LOSING WEIGHT
IS NOT ROCKET SCIENCE

Edward J. Walsh, Ph.D.

TOA PRESS LLC
Boulder, Colorado

LOSING WEIGHT IS NOT ROCKET SCIENCE

TOA PRESS LLC, P.O. Box 2262, Boulder, Colorado, 80306

ISBN-13: 978-0-9822989-1-6
ISBN-10: 0-9822989-1-9

CHAPTERS

1 INTRODUCTION

I'm going to tell you about the simplest and easiest way to lose weight, whether you have a lot to lose or just a little. And I'll show you what other books won't. How fast you can expect your weight to decrease. You can achieve your weight loss goal. You can feel better, have more confidence, improve your health, and your appearance.

More than a third of adults and 17% of youth in the United States are now obese according to the *Journal of the American Medical Association* (Ogden et al., 2014). But being overweight or obese is also a worldwide problem. An extensive analysis by 140 researchers (Ng et al., 2014) in the British medical journal *The Lancet* indicated that weight increased significantly between 1980 and 2013. Worldwide, 37% of men and 38% of women are now overweight or obese.

Weight also increased substantially in children and adolescents in developed countries with 24% of boys and

23% of girls overweight or obese in 2013. Overweight and obesity even increased in children and adolescents in developing countries, from 8% in 1980 to 13% in 2013 for both boys and girls. Adult obesity now exceeds 50% for men in Tonga and for women in Kuwait, Kiribati, Federated States of Micronesia, Libya, Qatar, Tonga and Samoa.

The good news is that, after having worked for NASA more than 40 years, I can assure you that losing weight is not rocket science. When I was 26 years old, I was New England Judo Champion and weighed 205 pounds. Ten years ago, when my weight hit an all-time high of 227 pounds, 22 pounds (10 kg) above my fighting weight, I decided to take action.

I had heard that marathon runners "hit the wall" when they've depleted the glycogen stored in their muscles from that big pasta meal the night before the race and have to burn fat, which the body doesn't want to do. It suddenly occurred to me that if you don't put any calories in your body for a 20-hour interval, it will have to burn fat. That may sound severe, but it is very effective and I'll explain why it's not difficult.

I did a two-year case study with daily weight measurements, from March 2004 through March 2006. Without changing my exercise routine or what I ate, my weight dropped 44 pounds, seamlessly transitioning into an ideal maintenance weight of 183 pounds and a Body Mass Index (BMI) of 23. That was 22 pounds below my fighting weight, but if you're not as strong as you were in your mid-twenties, you have less muscle mass and you should weigh less.

I initially called my technique **The Fast Way to Lose Weight** and submitted my results to the *American Journal of Bariatric Medicine*. Bariatricians are physicians who specialize in obesity. They published my article in the Fall of 2006, giving it top billing on the cover.

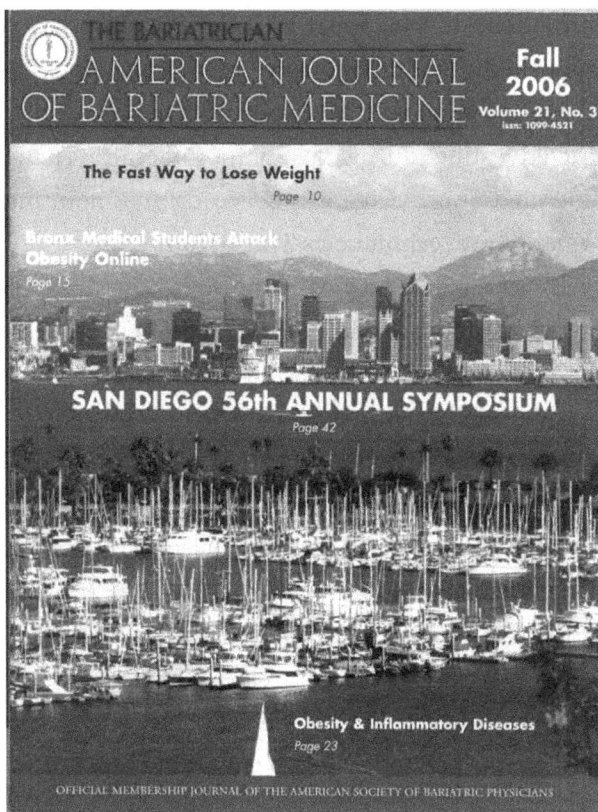

THE BARIATRICIAN
AMERICAN JOURNAL
OF BARIATRIC MEDICINE

Fall 2006
Volume 21, No. 3
issn: 1099-4521

The Fast Way to Lose Weight
Page 10

Bronx Medical Students Attack Obesity Online
Page 15

SAN DIEGO 56th ANNUAL SYMPOSIUM
Page 42

Obesity & Inflammatory Diseases
Page 23

OFFICIAL MEMBERSHIP JOURNAL OF THE AMERICAN SOCIETY OF BARIATRIC PHYSICIANS

My case study showed that you can live in the real world with all its disruptions and still attain your ideal weight. I retired from NASA in 2009 and, with time on my hands, expanded the analysis of my case study. On 23 September 2012, I published **Attain and Maintain your Ideal Weight**, my initial ebook describing the results of my weight-loss technique.

On 14 January 2013, Lorel Kelly, a knowledgeable friend in Connecticut, pointed out that **The 8-Hour Diet: Watch the Pounds Disappear Without Watching What You Eat!**, published three months after my book, had essentially the same technique. My case study had employed unrestricted eating during a 4-hour interval. Their book recommended unrestricted eating during an 8-hour interval. I now refer to my technique as **The 4-Hour Diet**.

There is a discrepancy in the authors and publication date of the hardbound edition of **The 8-Hour Diet** and the ebook. Amazon.com indicates the ebook was published on 24 December 2012 with authors David Zinczenko, Peter Moore and Matt Goulding. The hardbound edition has a 2013 copyright date by Rodale Inc. and indicates the author is David Zinczenko with Peter Moore. Matt Goulding is given one of the many acknowledgments.

I was surprised to find that more than half of **The 8-Hour Diet** was recipes and exercises. There may be foods that are better for you than some of the ones you're eating, but all those recipes seemed to be at odds with **The 8-Hour**

Diet subtitle, **Watch the Pounds Disappear Without Watching What You Eat!**

I looked over the Amazon customer reviews. What Amazon highlighted as **The most helpful favorable review** was a 5-star posting by **SS** on 30 December 2012. She gave a glowing endorsement to the book because "The author makes a simple, clear, compelling argument for intermittent fasting which I used successfully for nearly twenty years."

It was then I realized I had invented intermittent fasting. I just wasn't the first person to invent it, or the second, or third.

What Amazon highlighted as **The most helpful critical review** was a 3-star posting by B. Scott, also on 30 December 2012. Part of it said, "… 'The 8 Hour Diet' was [allegedly] stolen from leangains.com, Martin Berkhan's website. He has been writing about the 16/8 fasting diet for years, which in turn has turned the bodybuilding world upside down. He has changed countless amounts of blog and forum members lives with his methods. It's a shame 'The 8 Hour Diet' makes no mention of him or his website."

While preparing this introduction I become aware of **The Fast-5 Diet and the Fast-5 Lifestyle** by Bert W. Herring, M.D., which Amazon indicates was published on 28 October 2005, when I was about three quarters of the way through my two-year case study. It is nearly identical to my technique since Herring recommends unrestricted eating during a 5-hour interval instead of my 4-hour interval.

I'm not aware of anyone claiming that **The 8-Hour Diet** was copied from **The Fast-5 Diet**, but one of the Amazon 1-star reviews of **The Fast-5 Diet** posted by Erika Young on 29 July 2013 indicated that it "… is pretty much a copycat of "The warrior diet" by Ori Hofmekler which was published 2 years earlier 2003. The warrior diet and lifestyle is a superior book and is the original. I am tired of writers stealing other people's ideas and marketing them under new names."

That seems to be a theme of negative reviews of diet books. Different people can certainly conceive of the same thing independently. All books dealing with intermittent fasting have to be fundamentally the same: eat during a restricted time interval. David Zinczenko was the editor in chief of *Men's Health*, the editorial director of *Women's Health*, and the author of three other New York Times bestselling books on diet and health. You might assume he had to be aware of everything relating to health and diet but that is not necessarily the case.

I looked over the second edition of the **Warrior Diet**, published in 2007. Hofmekler has the least restrictive approach. He indicates that you should eat a meal only once a day, preferably at night, without any restriction on micronutrient content or calories. But he says that it is acceptable to nibble during the day as long as you exclude carbohydrates like grains and breads and snack on fruits, fresh vegetables, or a little protein.

Hofmekler is focused principally on how the ancient Greeks and Romans lived. Similar to **The 8-Hour Diet**, the **Warrior Diet** contains many recommendations for exercise, food and recipes. In contrast, Herring was a physician and **The Fast-5 Diet** is very different, mainly focused on how you can work your way into eating within a 5-hour window each day. Herring indicates that he first invented the technique in 1995, 8 years before the **Warrior Diet** was published, using motivation similar to mine.

I was amazed at the benefits **The 8-Hour Diet** ascribed to intermittent fasting: dramatically slash the risk of heart disease, diabetes and cancer; improve brain function, think more clearly; protect mind and body from the effects of stress and aging; significantly increase life expectancy and fight the inflammation at the heart of Alzheimer's. In the **Warrior Diet**, in addition to predicting similar general health benefits and suggesting that thoughts should become clearer and more focused, Hofmekler indicates that it can also enhance sex hormones.

Wow!!! If all that is true, you'll be even better off with my technique than theirs, but I'll get into that later.

If someone tells you that doing this or that will make the mitochondria in your cells burn fuel more efficiently, does that make the process work any better for you? It may increase your motivation to persevere if you believe that there is some scientific guarantee of success, but the process will either work or not work whether you are aware of the microbiological mechanisms or not.

Since my 20-hour fasting technique was developed independently, my analysis is very different from those other three books. None of them realistically indicate how you can expect your weight to vary. Improving what you eat and how much you exercise are certainly beneficial, but my graphs show you how you can expect your weight to vary if you change nothing but when you eat.

There is not a single graph in **The 8-Hour Diet**, **The Fast-5 Diet**, the **Warrior Diet**, nor any of the dozen other books I've looked through, to indicate how fast you can expect your weight to decrease. **The 8-Hour Diet** includes just 7 success stories, each with a single value of weight loss. One person reported losing 10 pounds in 4 weeks and 6 people indicated they lost 12 to 20 pounds in 6 weeks. The person losing 20 pounds weighed 315 pounds to begin with. Such snippets may help motivate people, but citing a single number is misleading because my graphs for **The 4-Hour Diet** show that weight loss is not linear and there is a significant initial weight loss over the first few days of fasting before the long-term trend is established.

In **The Fast-5 Diet**, Herring says that a pound a week is a reasonable weight loss goal. He indicates that you could maintain that rate of weight loss for a year – 52 pounds, if you have that much to lose. That is misleading because the rate of weight loss is not constant over that time span.

The graphs of daily weight variation from my case study and other medical research going back over 40 years indicate that you can expect an exponential decrease of your excess fat.

The daily weight measurements provide great insight and contrast the significant difference between weight fluctuations and body fat variation. The day to day fluctuations in your weight will always be large compared to the downward trend in your weight.

My graphs demonstrate why nobody should get discouraged by a large weight gain over a multiday period of non-adherence. Such gains do not indicate a large accumulation of fat. The weight gained will be quickly lost when you resume fasting and will not prevent you from attaining and maintaining your ideal weight.

It is now 10 years since I began my 2-year case study. In the 8 years since it ended I have intermittently fasted intermittently. My present weight is 186 pounds. The selfie on the back cover shows what that means. I don't have the muscle mass I did at 26, but I'm not doing bad for 72. **The 4-Hour Diet** is a long-term solution to being overweight.

Effective for any culture or ethnicity,

The 4-Hour Diet

can give the world a waistline!

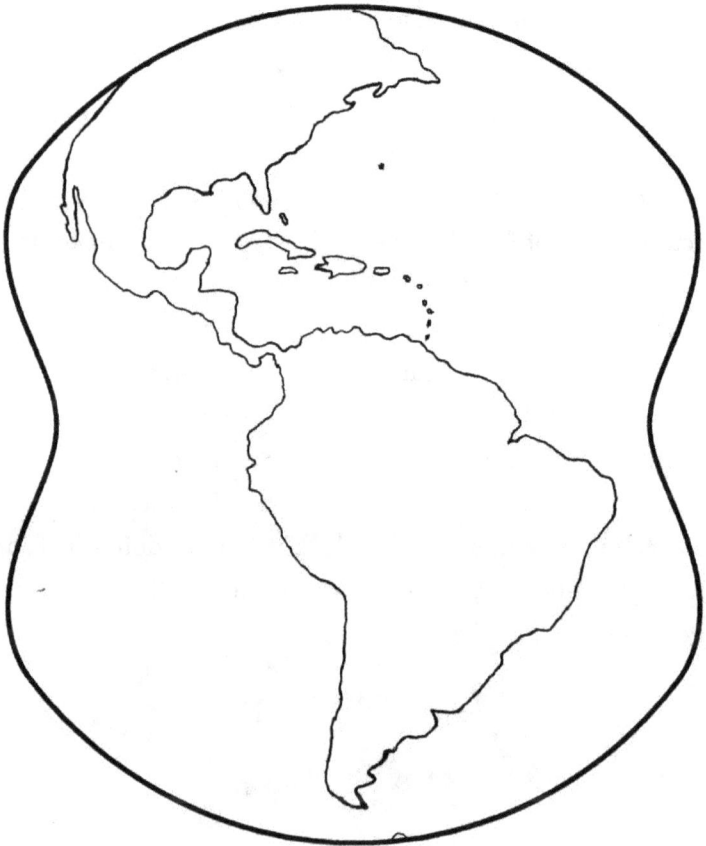

2 BACKGROUND

If you are not curious about my background, you can skip this chapter. In high school I wanted to be a musician. By eleventh grade I was lead trumpet in the band and orchestra and was in the Rhode Island Philharmonic Youth Orchestra. I also put together Ed's Clown Quartet to roam in and out stores playing Dixieland Jazz during Woonsocket's Mardi Gras celebration.

I planned to study trumpet at the New England Conservatory of Music, but fate took a turn. At the end of April the Woonsocket High orchestra played a two-night concert. The first night I cracked on a high C at the end of Carousel, which was embarrassing.

We had borrowed a French horn player from another school. His brother was lead trumpet in a South American symphony orchestra, so he had a lot of authority.

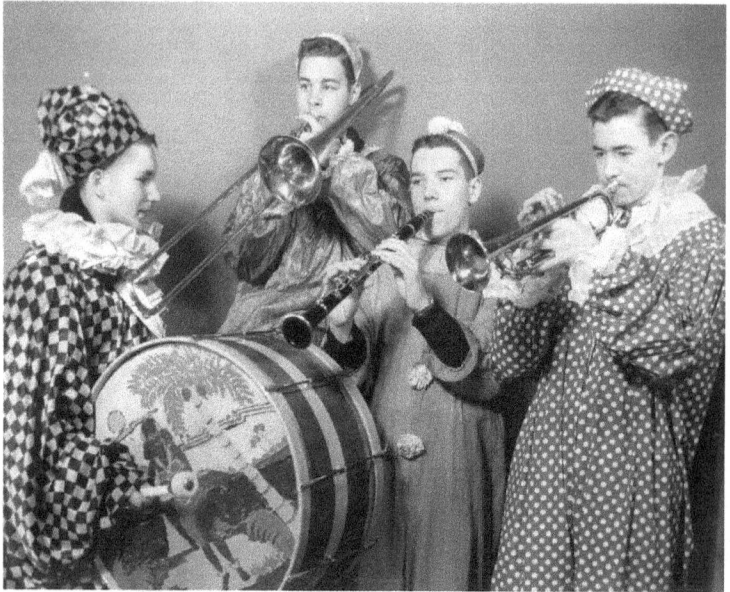

After the concert, he said I should tighten my belt and press very hard against it with my stomach to relieve the pressure on my lips so I wouldn't crack on the high C.

I did that the second night. The high C came out beautifully, but so did my guts. I got a strangulated hernia on that high C. I literally blew my guts out. Before the next song I whispered, "Roland, I've got a pain in my side."

"That's good, Ed. Shows you're using a lot of pressure."

The pain got worse as I played the rest of the concert. Roland whispered, "It's not supposed to hurt that much."

I had trouble walking up the aisle, but made it to a

drug store down the block and called my mother. Our family doctor managed to push the strangulation back inside so I wouldn't be rushed to the hospital. After corrective surgery a month later, the doctor told me not to play the trumpet for six months. I would not make the New England Conservatory audition.

My older brother was finishing freshman year in electrical engineering. "You're good at math. Electrical engineering is mostly math. Why not try that?" I studied hard senior year and got a scholarship to Northeastern University. By the time I graduated I was good at figuring things out, stuck around for a Ph.D., and went to work for NASA. Some years later they awarded me the NASA Medal for Exceptional Scientific Achievement.

Even though it was very painful, I now look back on that hernia fondly because it strangulated my musical career. I would have starved as a musician. I liked music but didn't have any real talent in it. In high school, being a good student can compensate for that.

From that and several other events in my life I realized two important things. First, it's frequently only possible to tell in retrospect whether something is actually good or bad. Second, your ultimate success or failure is more determined by how you respond to life's difficulties than by being lucky enough to avoid them.

Because of the trumpet and my hernia, I had never been involved with sports. In my third year of college I started playing judo. The photos show two of my trophies and me at 26 being congratulated by Harry Yanagi, the President of the New England Yudanshakai, United States Judo Federation (USJF), on my promotion to Nidan, Black Belt – Second Degree (USJF registration number 2-1184; Kodokan Judo Institute, Tokyo, registration number 1539), the same year I became New England Judo Champion.

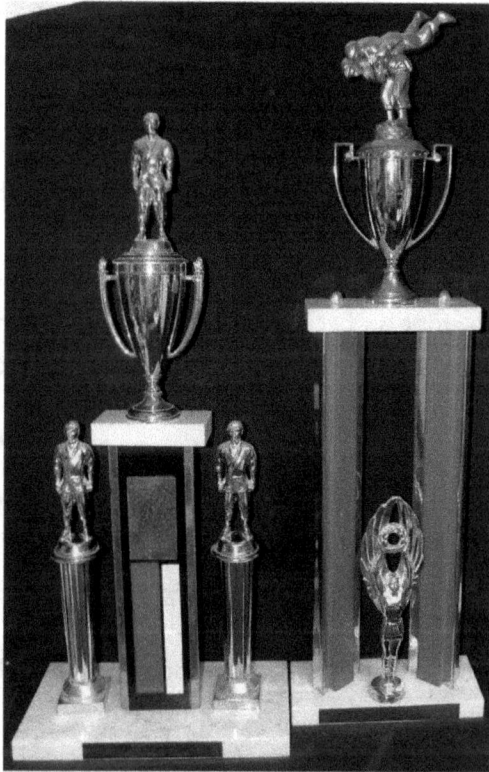

QUINCY Y JUDO CLUB
1ST SR INVIT NOV 12, 1967
OVERALL TOURNAMENT CHAMPION

4TH ANNUAL JOHN F. KENNEDY INV.
1967
GRAND CHAMPION

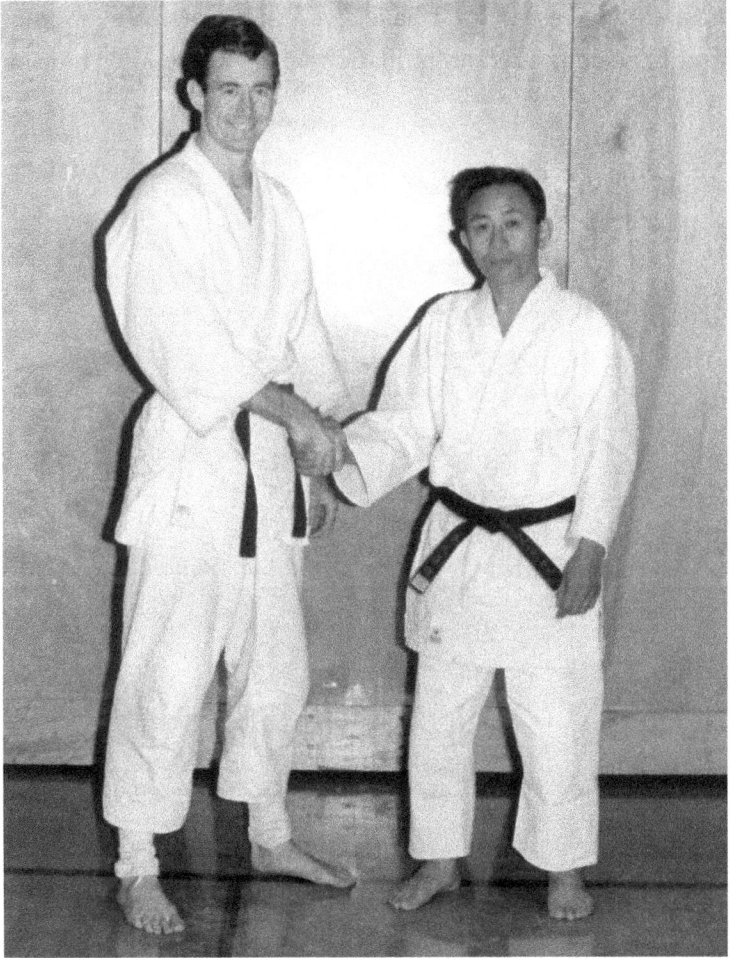

In 1982 the NASA/Goddard Space Flight Center in Maryland assigned me to what is now the National Oceanic and Atmospheric Administration (NOAA) Earth System Research Laboratory in Boulder, Colorado, to pursue cooperative research. I have lived in Colorado ever since and have continued an affiliation with NOAA after retiring from NASA.

3 WHY DON'T MOST DIETS WORK?

Why are most attempts to lose weight unsuccessful? Because people don't stick with whatever plan they select. When I decided to publish my case study I looked into the medical research on other weight loss programs and it was not encouraging.

A clinical trial published in the *Journal of the American Medical Association* (Dansinger et al., 2005) studied the **Adkins** (carbohydrate restriction), **Ornish** (fat restriction), **Weight Watchers** (calorie restriction), and **Zone** (macronutrient balance) diets. They started by screening over 1000 people by telephone, interviewed in person 247 of them who were overweight or obese, and then randomly assigned 40 of those to each of the four diets.

By the end of the year-long study, 14 to 20 people had dropped out of each diet, 42% of the participants on average, because they weren't able to stick it out. And the adherence of many of those who remained in the study decreased significantly during the year. Some participants did benefit, but, statistically, the diet type made little difference and all four failed because of low adherence and weight loss at 1 year.

One of the reasons so many people are used in clinical trials is to compensate for unreliable participants. If you start with many people and randomly divide them into four groups, you should statistically have the same ratio of conscientious to lackadaisical people in each group. You have to rely on the participants to characterize their own adherence and you want to have the same percentage of people in all groups who will exaggerate their effort.

If you include many people, you can have confidence that the best performing group will indicate the most effective technique either because the composition of that diet is most effective or it produces the highest adherence. The Adkins, Ornish, Weight Watchers, and Zone diets may be equally effective if followed, but the Dansinger et al. (2005) study indicated that typical people won't adhere to any of them for a year.

A different clinical trial, published in the *New England Journal of Medicine* (Wadden et al., 2005), used various combinations of medication and life-style modification counseling in group therapy sessions or delivered by a primary care provider. They started with about 240 people and randomly divided them into 4 groups.

One of the four groups was just given medication

(Sibutramine), a second group just attended intensive group therapy sessions on lifestyle modification. The third group got medication and brief counseling from the physician. The fourth group got the medication and the intensive group therapy sessions (combined therapy). The results are shown in Figure 1.

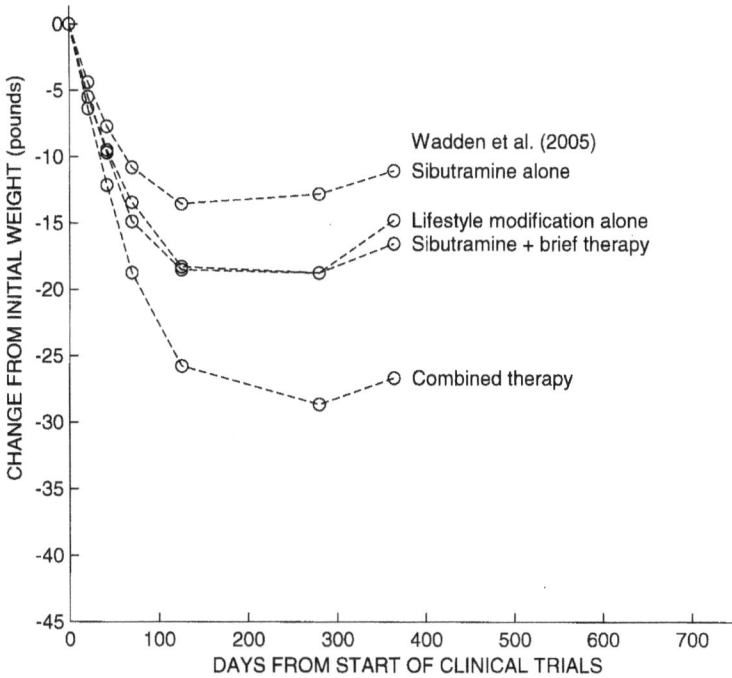

Figure 1

By the end of the Wadden et al. (2005) clinical trial the fourth group (combined therapy) had lost the most weight, indicating that the technique using medication coupled with intensive group therapy sessions was the most effective. But I think it's more significant that Figure 1 shows weight loss had bottomed out and weight was increasing for all four groups by the end of the one-year study. I'll bet most of the people were back up near where they began by the end of a second year.

Although I documented my weight on a nearly daily basis for my 2-year case study, in Figure 2 below I smoothed those values, over a month for day 16 and beyond, to make it easier to contrast with the Wadden et al. (2005) study. The thick curve shows that instead of starting back up after 9 months, I continued to lose weight and seamlessly transitioned into an ideal maintenance weight without making any adjustments to what I did.

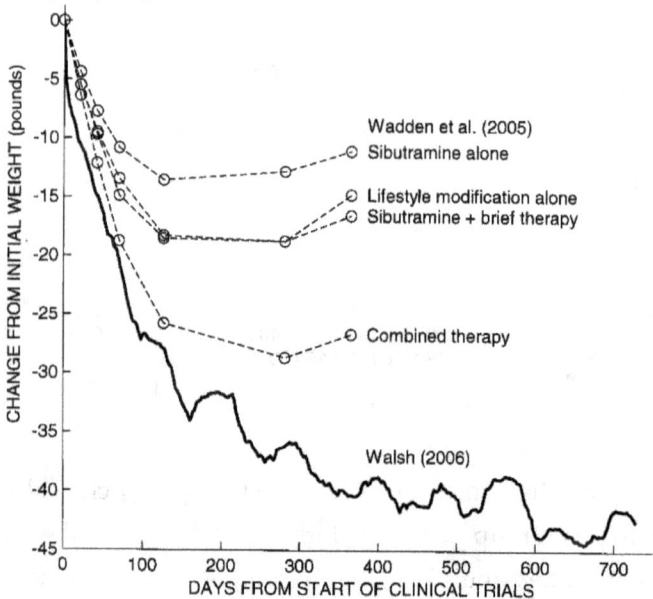

Figure 2

4 WHAT ABOUT EXERCISE?

Exercise is good, but eating can overwhelm it. That's obvious when you look at sumo wrestlers. You can also look closer to home. In the health club, I see guys with big biceps and bigger bellies.

I exercise more than most people, but that doesn't matter and it shouldn't concern you. I gave up judo after I got married, but I still ran. Back in 2000 my knees started bothering me. A surgeon at the Steadman-Hawkins Clinic in Vail, Colorado, told me I had a torn meniscus in both knees and the left was worse than the right. Fortunately, he was getting married shortly. He prescribed medication and scheduled my surgery for 6 weeks later.

The most important thing he told me was that running was bad for your knees because of the impact. After the medication made my knees feel better, I began walking on a treadmill and weaned myself from the medication. I never did have the surgery.

The plots in Figure 3 below show my treadmill activity and weight variation. I decided to walk on the treadmill for 36 minutes each time. I began doing about two and a half miles once or twice a week with a 10% incline. Over about a year and a half, I worked up to 3 miles at a 12% grade and generally did that 6 or 7 times a week.

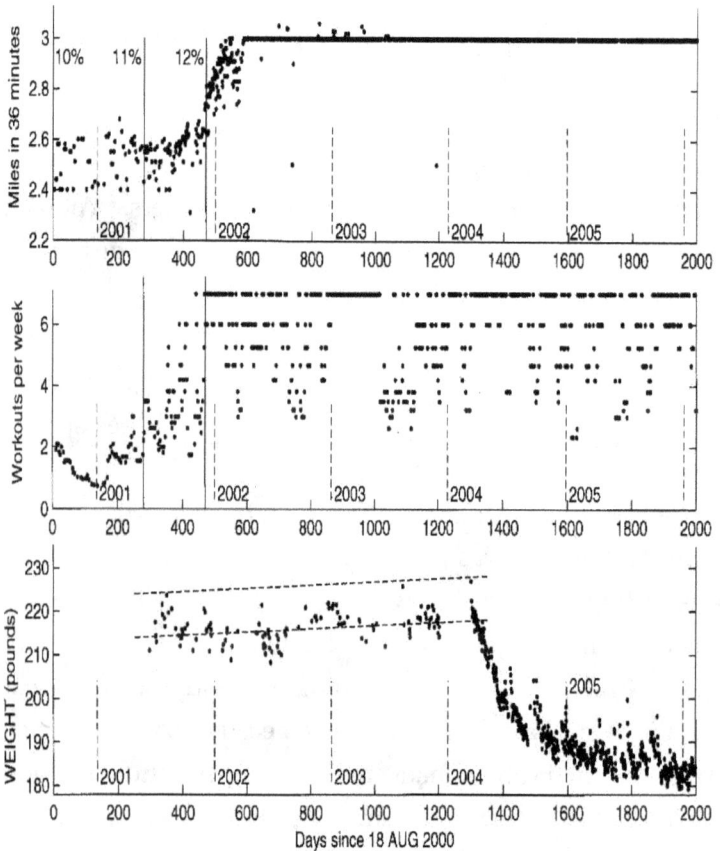

Figure 3

I didn't measure my weight routinely until I started my weight-loss case study. The occasional weights I did record fluctuated a lot. I least-squares fitted the lower dashed line through them to determine the general trend. It indicated that I was gaining about one and a third pounds a year. That may sound small, but at that rate I would be 20 pounds heavier in 15 years.

The upper dashed line in Figure 3 is just offset 10 pounds above the least-squares fitted dashed line to emphasize that my three high weights had been following the same increasing trend as the rest. I think that's how a lot of people put on weight as they age. Just little bit by little bit. Hardly noticeable until one day they wonder, How did I get so fat?

All that exercise was certainly benefitting my cardio-vascular state, but I was not losing weight. On 8 March 2004, my weight hit an all-time high of 227 pounds. I decided to take action and the plot shows the result. My exercise routine had been in steady state for a couple of years, so it was not responsible for my dramatic 44 pound weight loss.

5 HOW DO YOU GET RID OF FAT?

As you consider my weight-loss technique you need to keep in mind that I'm not a physician. I want to help you, but my daughter was concerned that someone reading this will do something foolish, blame me, and file a lawsuit. So I need to make a strong disclaimer.

This book does not constitute medical advice. You are strongly encouraged to consult your physician prior to beginning this technique to be certain you have no medical or mental condition that might contraindicate my suggestions, which are for educational purposes and not intended to substitute for your health care provider. Any product names or trademarks are assumed to be the property of their respective owners and are used only for reference. The mention of any individual or organization is for informational purposes only and does not imply any endorsement of them or by them.

Readers must rely on their own judgment regarding their circumstances and limitations, act accordingly and take full responsibility for their own safety. The purchaser or reader of this book assumes full responsibility for the use of this information and I and my publisher assume no liability or responsibility whatsoever on behalf of any purchaser or reader of this material.

There is no guarantee of results. Nothing in this book is intended to replace common sense or appropriate or necessary medical advice or care. Do not follow any recommendation that contradicts your physician's advice. My publisher and I disclaim any liability or loss, personal or otherwise, resulting from the information in this book.

Some of my information is garnered from the world wide web and personal interactions so its accuracy isn't guaranteed. I'll tell you what I did and why I believe it works. My weight loss numbers are accurate, but if you have any concerns about my analysis or interpretation of the numbers, consult your own physician.

The 4-Hour Diet can be stated very concisely.
Fast 20 hours a day.
> **If you go to bed at 10 PM,**
>> **no calories before 6 PM,**
>> **unrestricted eating after 6 PM.**

This is an incredibly simple way to implement the obvious solution to being overweight. If you eat less, you will weigh less. With fasting you don't have to change what you eat or give up the foods you love. You don't have to eat foods you don't love. You don't have boxes of food showing up on your doorstep. There is no bookkeeping. It costs nothing to fast. You'll even save money by not having to buy lunch.

There may be some foods that would be better for you than the ones you're eating. But if you just eat less of the ones you like, you will lose weight. When you do eat, you can eat until you're full rather than having to deprive yourself.

I believe that if you do what I did, you will attain your ideal weight, as I did. But I want to make sure you understand what I mean by unrestricted eating after 6 PM. I never worried about what I ate and I did not change the composition of my diet when I began fasting. I ate the same foods I had always eaten. **The 4-Hour Diet** simply reduced the amount I ate of them.

Suppose you made a detailed list of everything you consumed during a week. In the second week you fast until 6 PM each day and then place everything you had consumed during that day the previous week on a table. You could eat whatever you wanted during the next 4 hours, but you would not finish it all.

Fasting 20 hours a day will effectively reduce the quantity of the food you had been eating and you will lose weight. If you also improve the composition of your diet you will do even better than I did, but that is not necessary to achieve my results. If you use "unrestricted eating after 6 PM" as a license to seriously degrade your diet, you will not do as well.

The 8-Hour Diet and the **Warrior Diet** go to great lengths to encourage you to improve the composition of your diet and increase the amount of exercise you do. One of the most severe weight loss programs I've looked at is **SHRED: THE REVOLUTIONARY DIET** by Ian Smith, M.D. (2013). On page 2 he indicates that the average weight loss over his 6-week program for the hundreds of people who provided feedback was between 18 and 25 pounds. Losing 25 pounds in 6 weeks is almost double the initial loss rate of **The 4-Hour Diet**. But with **SHRED** you must eat highly specified foods in highly restricted quantities at 7 highly specified times each day and do a minimum of 30 to 45 minutes of cardiovascular exercise five days a week. While effective, it might be difficult for most people to reorient their lives and disrupt their normal activities to that extent. Since Smith has written several bestselling diet books and has over 48,000 twitter followers, hundreds or even thousands of people saying they have succeeded is a small subset of those who have tried his program. It is important to find a program you can stick with.

The 4-Hour Diet would be effective for any culture or ethnic group since it results in you eating less of the foods you normally eat. People talk about inner city food deserts causing obesity because of the lack of wholesome food. Improving the composition of a bad diet would reduce obesity, but so would decreasing the amount you consume of the foods available to you.

I believe my twenty-hour fasting technique is easier to adhere to than any diet program. There are no distractions, no particular foods to prepare and have available, no requirement throughout the day to remember what you need to eat and when you need to eat it.

My data show that if you fast most days, the occasions when you do not fast will not matter and the weight you gain will be quickly lost when you resume fasting.

Why is adherence easier with **The 4-Hour Diet**?

When you eat, your blood sugar elevates. Then you get hunger pangs when your blood sugar drops. If you eat breakfast, your stomach will empty out by noon. Your elevated blood sugar will drop and you'll be hungry for lunch. When you eat lunch, your stomach will empty out by 6 PM, your blood sugar will drop, and you'll be hungry for dinner.

You're asleep when your blood sugar drops during the night so you don't get hunger pangs. It's low when you get up in the morning. If you don't consume any calories before 6 PM, you will not get hunger pangs because your blood sugar will just stay low.

In the 4 hours of unrestricted eating after 6 PM your stomach will be capacity-limited. You can eat until you're full and you will consume less food than you would have distributed throughout the day.

The 4-Hour Diet is also an effective way to eliminate the weight gain associated with emotional eating. Without realizing it, you may have been eating comfort food during the day to get relief from stress, frustration, or anxiety. Maybe you were bored or depressed. Or angry, lonely, or thought you weren't worthwhile.

With **The 4-Hour Diet** you can't fool yourself. Fasting is an absolute. You can't tell yourself "That candy bar didn't have that many calories" or "I'll only eat a small piece of the cake." You're either fasting or you're not fasting. There are no degrees of compliance.

Before I began my case study, if I ate something for breakfast I'd be very distracted by hunger by 11 AM and go to the cafeteria to get some chocolate covered donuts. Now, a chocolate sheet cake in the copy room doesn't tempt me. It's far easier to eat nothing than to eat a little and stop. Don't jack up your blood sugar.

During my 2-year case study there were times when I began eating at 5 PM instead of 6 PM, and other times when I didn't begin eating until 7 or 8 PM. But 6 PM was by far the most frequent time I began eating and it is the appropriate time to use in evaluating the effectiveness of the technique.

It is interesting that **The 8-Hour Diet** extensively references Mark P. Mattson, Ph.D., a researcher at the National Institute on Aging and a Professor in the Department of Neuroscience at the Johns Hopkins

University School of Medicine. The **Warrior Diet** also references him. What does Dr. Mattson do that he believes is optimum? "Skip breakfast and lunch and exercise instead, then eat a nice meal over dinner." Sounds like **The 4-Hour Diet** to me.

There were days when I didn't fast at all and just pigged out. I will discuss them and their effect in detail so you can see that such lapses will not thwart your goals.

6 INSULIN AND FAT LOSS

Insulin is a storage hormone that regulates blood sugar by moving the sugar from the blood into the liver and muscles to be readily available for use and converting any excess to fat for a reserve. If you eat foods throughout the day that are high in sugar or starch that is converted to sugar, you won't be able to access and burn your fat reserves because your insulin level will remain high, keeping you in fat storage mode.

David S. Ludwig, M.D., Ph.D., is a professor of pediatrics at Harvard Medical School and directs the New Balance Foundation Obesity Prevention Center at Boston Children's Hospital.   Mark I. Friedman, Ph.D., is vice president of research at the Nutrition Science Initiative in San Diego.

Ludwig and Friedman (2014) reported that a nation-wide survey indicated only one in six overweight or obese adults ever maintained a 10% weight loss for a year. And they thought even that modest success rate was probably exaggerated because people tend to overestimate their accomplishments when self-reporting.

They indicated that some obesity researchers believe people have a body weight set point that is predetermined by their genes. That theory can't explain the obesity epidemic in the U.S. because the gene pool doesn't change much in a generation or two and the adult obesity rate is now almost three times what it was in the 1960s. So the good news is that most people who are overweight today were not predestined to be fat.

Ludwig and Friedman acknowledged that genetics is one of many biological factors affecting the storage of calories in fat cells, in addition to physical activity, sleep and stress. But they emphasized that it is the insulin hormone that has the indisputable dominant role in increasing fat. When treating diabetes, insulin deficiency causes weight loss and excess insulin causes weight gain.

Ludwig and Friedman suggested that the obesity increase has occurred because, starting in the 1970s, many refined carbohydrates have been added to processed foods to replace fats in the American diet. The resulting increase in insulin levels has put fat cells into storage overdrive. But **The 4-Hour Diet** can greatly improve your situation no matter what you have been eating.

Insulin variation throughout the day has been well documented for two different diets, high-starch and high-sucrose, in a British medical research paper published in the **American Journal of Clinical Nutrition**. The Daly et al. (1998) study at the University of Newcastle upon Tyne, United Kingdom, involved eight healthy adults (four men and four women, average age 25, ranging from 20 to 31). Insulin levels for each subject were measured during two 24-hour periods while they were receiving high-starch and high-sucrose diets.

The study was a randomized crossover design such that four of the participants received the high-sucrose diet first and the other four received the high-starch diet first. The two study periods were separated by at least one week for the men and one month for the women to keep as close as possible to a fixed point in their menstrual cycles.

Four meals were served using the following percentage distribution of the total food energy for the day: breakfast (18%) at 8 AM, lunch (35%) at noon, dinner (34%) at 5 PM, and supper (13%) at 8 PM. Water was allowed freely during the study period and one cup of tea or instant decaffeinated coffee was allowed with each meal.

Twenty-seven blood samples were taken each day, at 30-minute intervals for 2 hours after each of the meals, then hourly except every two hours overnight. The group average insulin variations resulting from the two types of meals are shown in Figure 4. Insulin rose more rapidly to a higher peak value with the high-sucrose diet, but then fell below the high-starch diet one to two hours later.

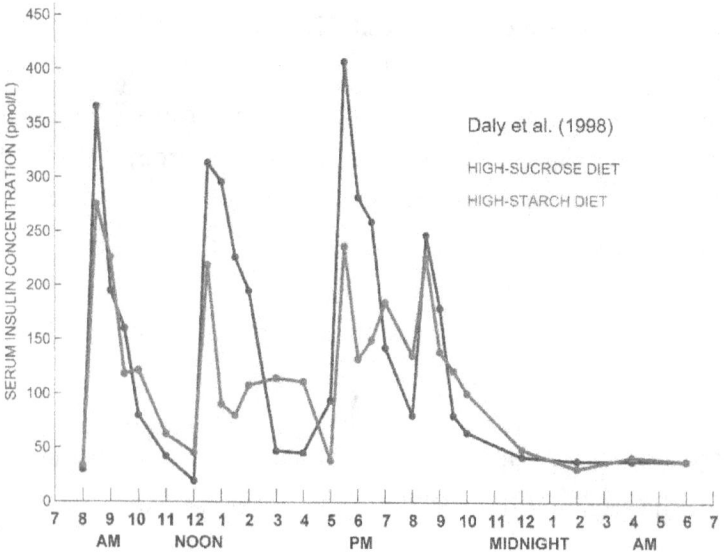

Figure 4

The food in the study was very tightly controlled with each item weighed to the nearest 0.1 g (0.004 ounce) during meal preparation. If the participants had been allowed to snack between meals, they might never have achieved a low insulin level while they were awake.

Because the participants fasted from 10 PM the night before each day of the study, the Daly et al. (1998) data can be used to estimate the variation of insulin for someone using **The 4-Hour Diet**. In Figure 5, the insulin level from Figure 4 for the high-starch diet at 5 PM was used as a starting point, but shifted to 6 PM, the nominal starting time of **The 4-Hour Diet** unrestricted eating interval.

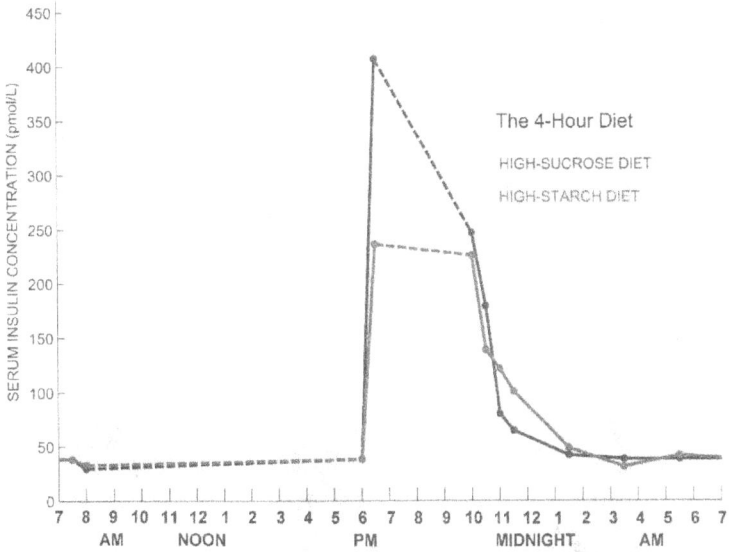

Figure 5

The next points were the 5:30 PM values from Figure 4, shifted to 6:30 PM in Figure 5. Those peak insulin values were then connected by dashed lines to the 8:30 PM values from Figure 4 which were shifted to 10 PM in Figure 5, the nominal ending time of the 4-hour interval of unrestricted eating. The remaining values from 9 PM through 6 AM in Figure 4 were then plotted in Figure 5, but shifted forward by an hour and a half. Dashed lines connect the 8 AM values from Figure 4 and the 6 PM values in Figure 5.

There would probably be insulin oscillations in the dashed region of Figure 5 from 6:30 PM through 10 PM, depending on what was consumed during that interval. But

Figure 5 indicates that insulin would be at a minimum level more than 16 hours each day for someone using **The 4-Hour Diet**.

THE FAST WAY TO LOSE WEIGHT

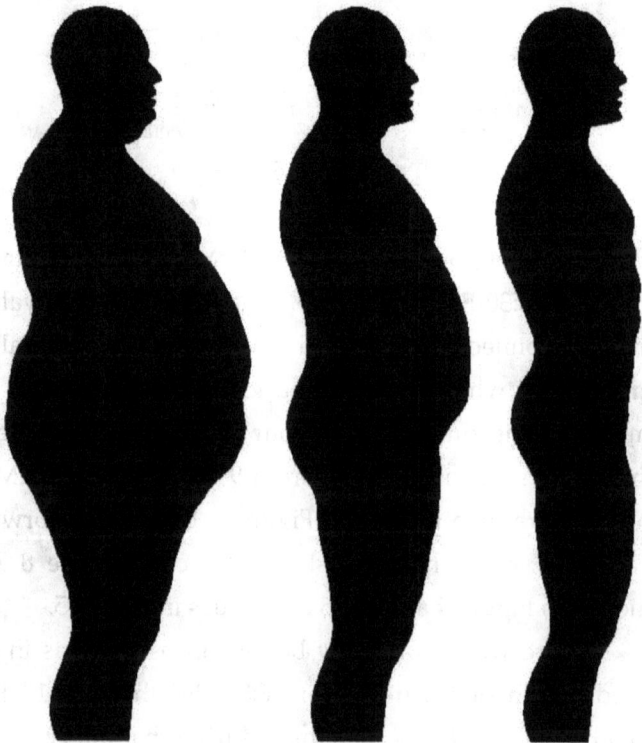

7 ISN'T IS BAD TO EAT IN THE EVENING?

Melina Jampolis, M.D., a nutrition specialist and author of **The No-Time to Lose Diet: The Busy Person's Guide to Permanent Weight Loss** (2007) said, "There is nothing unique about eating too many calories after 8 PM. This just happens to be the time that people snack mindlessly on chips and dessert while watching TV."

Some weight-loss "experts" recommend not eating after 7 or 8 PM because eliminating late-night snacking will reduce total caloric intake if you have been eating during the day. Dr. Jampolis indicated that there's nothing different about the way your body handles calories in the evening. Calories consumed late in the day will not generate more fat than calories consumed early in the day.

However, telling people not to snack may be why many people don't stick to any diet. Most people work hard during the day and just want to relax and enjoy themselves at night. If you tell them they can't enjoy a snack as they visit with friends and family or watch T.V., they may feel frustrated and deprived and give up trying to lose weight altogether.

Since it doesn't matter when you consume your calories, fasting during the day allows you to eat as much as you want at night without guilt. When I started to fast, the first couple of days I ate to the point of discomfort at night ("I can't believe I ate the whole thing.") and still lost weight rapidly.

8   WILL YOUR BODY GO INTO
STARVATION MODE?

My weight measurements demonstrate that my body did not go into starvation mode, significantly reducing my metabolism and preventing me from losing weight. It takes much longer than 20 hours of fasting for your body to shut down your metabolism. Some people might consider that statement to be against the conventional wisdom.

For example, on 26 August 2012, *Parade Magazine* quoted *The Biggest Loser* trainer Bob Harper as saying, "So many people think skipping breakfast will help them lose. I've been in the health business for over 20 years, and I've seen how much that can slow down your metabolism."

I don't believe it. Harper's belief may be the result of a possible side effect of my fasting technique. During my rapid weight loss phase, I occasionally noticed a reduced alertness in the afternoon during fasting if I was just sitting at my desk and not physically active. On those occasions I might not have gotten enough rest the night before. But it is possible that, like the marathon runners "hitting the wall" when their bodies are burning fat, that inefficient process of metabolizing fat reduces the amount of energy you have and makes you want to nap. Heavy equipment operators should exercise caution.

I've heard a lot of people say that when they need to get something done in a hurry they eat a candy bar to get a sugar high. Your body would much prefer burning a candy bar to burning fat, which is its reserve and security blanket. A little lethargy, which some people think indicates a significant decrease in metabolism that will thwart your weight loss goals, might actually indicate you are burning fat and achieving your weight loss goals.

9 INSIGHTS PROVIDED BY A DAILY WEIGHT RECORD

During my research at NASA I learned that very detailed observations can lead to great insights. Once I began fasting, I recorded my weight prior to working out nearly every day, when I was not traveling. I always used one of two good quality scales that I cross-calibrated on numerous occasions. One was at the health club and the other was at work. I also subtracted the weight of whatever clothes I was wearing. I was very careful with the measurements and I am confident that my weights are accurate to better than a quarter pound. I did not record my weight when I was traveling because those scales could not be cross-calibrated.

The circles in Figure 6 below show my weight variation over the first 120 days of my case study. The diameter of the circles in that plot and the next three showing my weight variation over the two-year case study is less than 1 pound. Since I believe the error in my weights is less than a quarter pound, any variation you notice in the sequence of weights is a real change in my weight, not a measurement error.

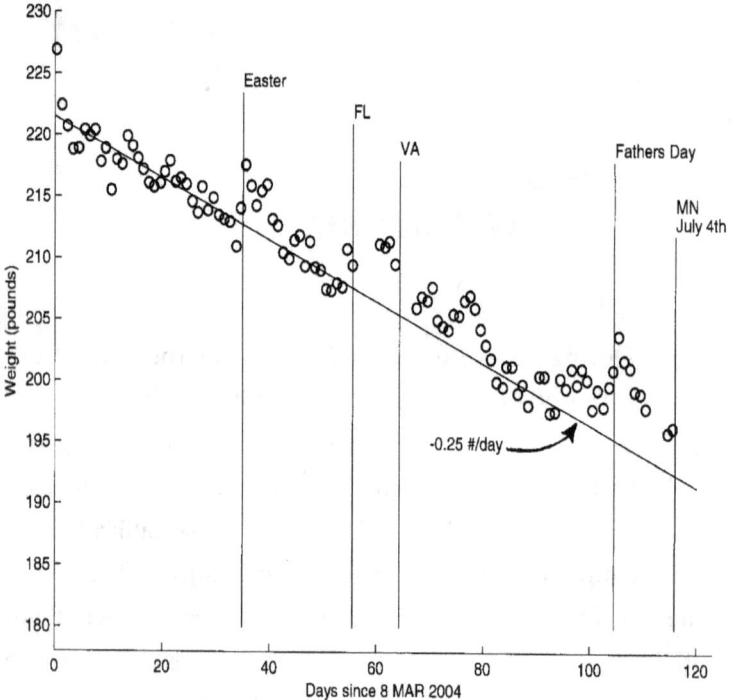

Figure 6

The straight line in Figure 6 is not least-squares fitted to the data but is just drawn to indicate a constant rate of decrease of a quarter pound each day. It well represents the average rate of weight loss over the first 100 days. Every four days I lost a pound of fat, on average. What is the volume of a pound of fat? Look at a pound of butter.

42

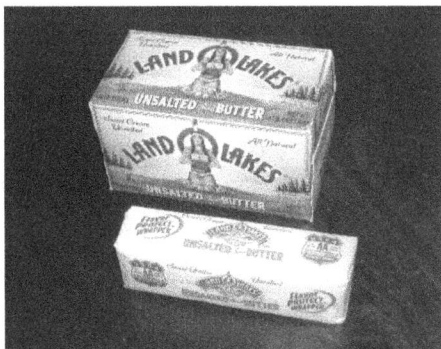

If you rapidly lost several pounds of fat right from where you buckle your belt, that would be really impressive. But that's not what happens. For years I've heard trainers say that you can't "spot reduce" fat. If you want to get rid of the fat at a particular location you need to suck it out with liposuction. During dieting, the fat you lose leaches little by little from all over your body so the result is less noticeable in the short term.

My weight dropped almost 5 pounds the first day. The graph shows that my weight could also jump up 5 to 7 pounds in 2 or 3 days. Those were actual changes in my weight, not errors in the measurement. But what did they mean? To put the weight fluctuations in perspective I came up with the concept of "intrinsic" weight.

Suppose you weigh yourself, drink a bottle of water, and weigh yourself again. The scale will indicate that your weight has increased a pound. But your "intrinsic" weight hasn't changed at all. The scale would have told you the same thing if you had stuck the bottle in your pocket. You didn't consume any calories and you have the same amount of fat and muscle and bones as you did before you drank the water.

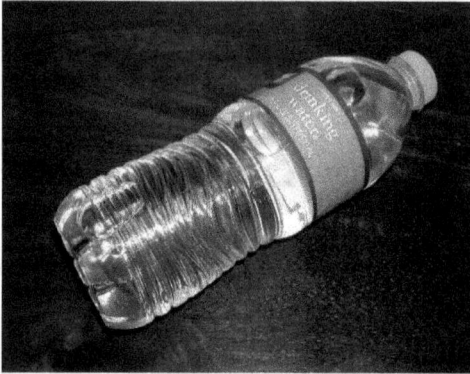

Suppose you weighed yourself in the morning and then didn't drink anything all day. Even though a scale would indicate you weighed a lot less at the end of the day, your intrinsic weight would not have decreased much. Becoming dehydrated is unhealthy and doesn't decrease your intrinsic weight. And drinking lots of water doesn't increase it.

If you are like most people, you eat throughout the day and your digestive track is filled and in steady state. When you start fasting, you disrupt that process. You don't put any food in your digestive track for 20 hours and a bunch of what was in there moves out, producing a significant weight drop.

I've heard some quick-loss diets boast that you can lose 5 pounds by the weekend. That may be useful in motivating people, but they are not losing 5 pounds of fat. In the first few days, your weight loss may seem to be from your beltline because that's where your intestines are. After that initial excitement your progress will be less apparent on a daily basis.

When I started to analyze the variation of my weight I noticed large fluctuations that were superimposed on the general decreasing trend. I have tried to identify significant events that had disrupted my fasting. The vertical lines on Figure 6 indicate 5 such events I identified during the first 4 months. In two days my weight increased about 7 pounds at Easter and 5 pounds at Father's Day. The other 3 vertical lines indicate when I left for business trips to Florida and Virginia and a vacation in Minnesota. The data gaps after those 3 lines indicate the length of the trip because I didn't record my weight while traveling.

Anybody trying to lose weight will have disruptions in their activities that will cause periods of non-adherence to whatever program they select. It's not reasonable to fast during family activities such as Easter and Father's Day, but the biggest disruptions during my case study were my wife's 4th of July family reunions in Minnesota and hurricanes.

From 1998 through 2005 I operated my NASA Scanning Radar Altimeter (SRA) on one of the NOAA hurricane research aircraft. The aircraft are named after Jim Henson's Muppets. The two WP-3D 4-engine turboprop aircraft (N42RF and N43RF) are Kermit and Miss Piggy and the Gulfstream G-IV jet aircraft (N49RF) is Gonzo. There is a special image of Miss Piggy in a flight suit with the words *Aero-Nautical ... But Nice!* just to the left of the entrance to N43RF, welcoming people to the aircraft.

Every morning during hurricane season there would be a teleconference. When a decision was made to fly, I'd have to get on a 6 PM flight out of Denver that arrived in Tampa, Florida, near midnight for a hurricane flight out of the NOAA Aircraft Operations Center the next morning. The pictures below show me sitting at the SRA controls and at the entrance to Miss Piggy.

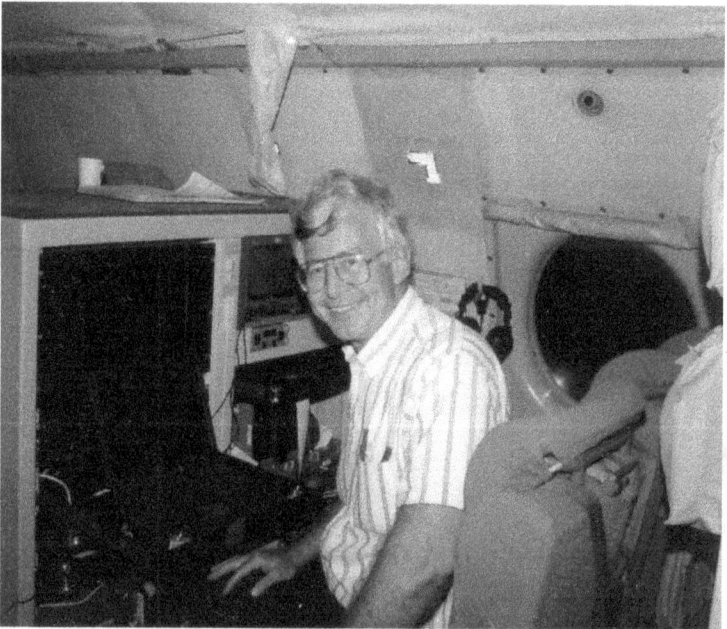

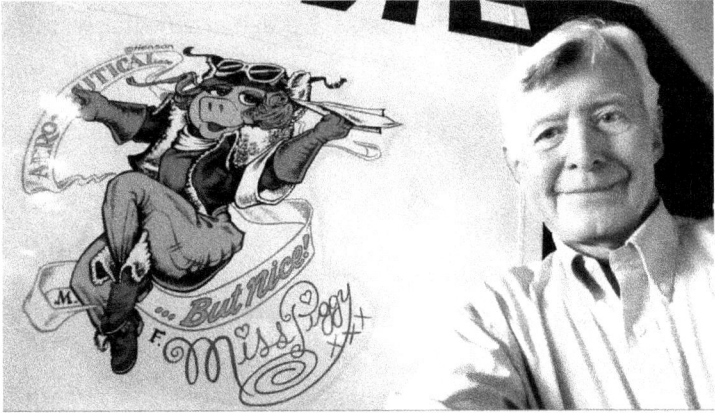

The flights generally lasted about 9 hours. We'd fly straight through the hurricane, in one side and out the other, at a height of 5,000 to 10,000 feet, depending on its strength. Then we'd fly around the outside to get to a new starting point and fly straight through it again and again until we ran out of time.

We wore heavy web shoulder straps that locked into our heavier web seat belts and things could get pretty bumpy going through the rain bands and the eyewall. But whenever we broke through into the eye, things immediately got peaceful. Sometimes the pilot would fly circles in the eye to give everybody time to use the single toilet before plunging back into the storm.

On the satellite image below, I have superimposed our flight path through Hurricane Katrina when it was Category 5 on 28 August 2005. The flight line begins at the NOAA Aircraft Operations Center at MacDill Air Force Base

in Tampa, Florida, and ends as we exited Katrina heading
back home.

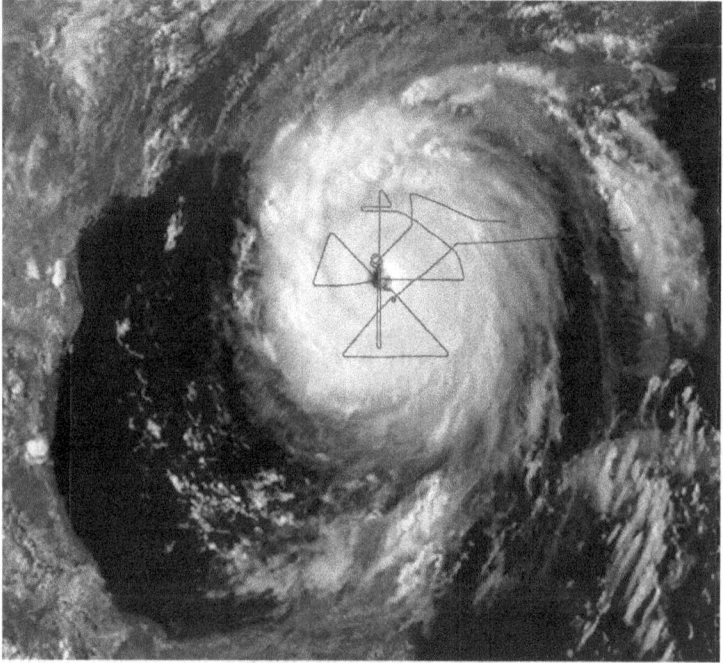

The satellite image of Katrina was acquired about
halfway through our flight. The eye location in the image
and the earlier and later eye locations, indicated by the
sequence of aircraft circles, show Katrina was turning North
towards New Orleans during our flight.

I've put two pictures below that I took out my
window at an altitude of 10,000 feet. Hurricane eyewalls
generally tilt outward as they go up. With the deep blue
cloudless sky above us, the Katrina eyewall on 28 August

2005 was brilliant white in the sunlight and gave the impression of a huge celestial amphitheater. There were gray swirls of clouds below us and between them you could see right down to the big waves Katrina was generating in the Gulf of Mexico.

The sun was in a different position when I took the picture of Rita's eyewall on 22 September 2005. It looked more like a dark wall rising up through the solid white cloud deck beneath us. To know more about the hurricane flights, get **Inside the Hurricane** by Pete Davies (2000).

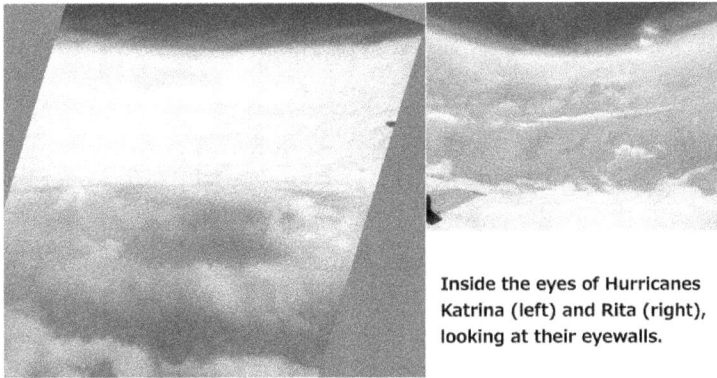

Inside the eyes of Hurricanes Katrina (left) and Rita (right), looking at their eyewalls.

Figure 7 shows my weight variation during days 112 through 273 of my case study, which overlaps a little with the end of the previous graph showing the first 120 days. Figure 7 indicates I put on about 11 pounds over the 4th of July in Minnesota. My wife is the 8th of 15 children and about 100 people gather at the lake home of one of her sisters in Minnesota over that long weekend. Eating is almost continuous with all the fun and great food.

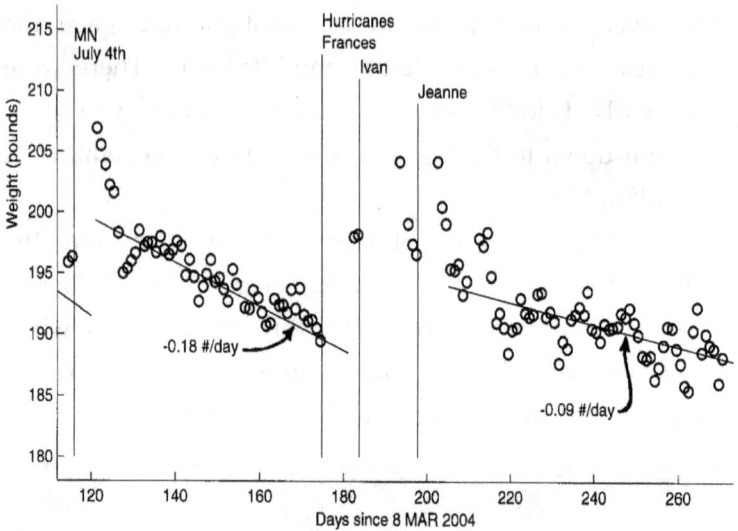

Figure 7

My weight recovered within a week of being back home and I was losing about 0.18 pound of fat per day over the next 50 days, reaching a new low of about 190 pounds, before I had to run to fly Hurricane Frances. My hurricane schedule was always hectic both pre- and post-flight. I never even tried fasting. Whenever we weren't strapped in our seats, I'd be munching on finger food in the Hog's Breath Café, the small galley area at the rear of Miss Piggy.

Figure 7 shows that I had put on about 8 pounds by the time I came back from Hurricane Frances and was home only two days before going back to Tampa for Hurricane Ivan. I came back from Ivan about an additional 7 pounds heavier. I dropped almost 8 pounds in a few days before returning to Tampa for Hurricane Jeanne, and I popped back up to my post-Ivan weight. Hurricane Jeanne was my last flight of the 2004 season.

Within a week back home I dropped about 10 pounds. Then my weight loss rate stabilized at about 0.09 pound of fat a day over the last two months of the plot. But even in that two-month interval when there were no major disruptive events, my weight could decrease or increase 6 or 7 pounds over the course of a week. Those fluctuations in weight were large, but they were not variations in fat. The straight lines much better represent how my fat content was varying over time, as I will discuss later.

Figure 8 shows my weight variation from day 267 through day 456. During this 6-month period my fat content was dropping by about 0.05 pound per day. That's only 0.8 ounce per day, but it was still dropping. It is important to keep in mind that my weight at the beginning of this interval was already down about 38 pounds from where I started. I had already accomplished almost all of my goal and was solidifying my much improved status. Contrast that with the weights of all four groups in the Wadden clinical trial (Figure 1), which were increasing at the start of this interval.

Even though my weight could jump up 7 to 10 pounds in a few days because of trips or holidays, as soon as I went back to fasting I shed the extra weight quickly because it was not fat. A significant part of those weight gains was my digestive track filling up and expanding. As it emptied back out, my weight dropped.

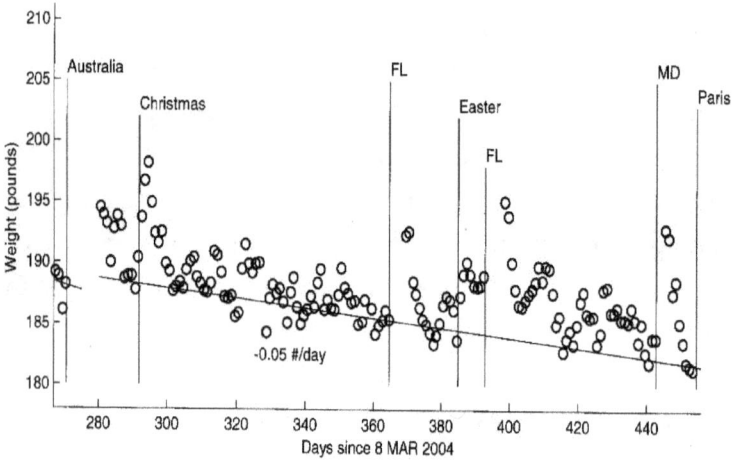

Figure 8

Figure 9 shows my weight variation over days 450 through 680. By the end of that interval my weight had stabilized and I was no longer losing fat. I was surprised that I put on about 17 pounds in Minnesota over the 4th of July that year, but after a couple of weeks of fasting my weight was right back down.

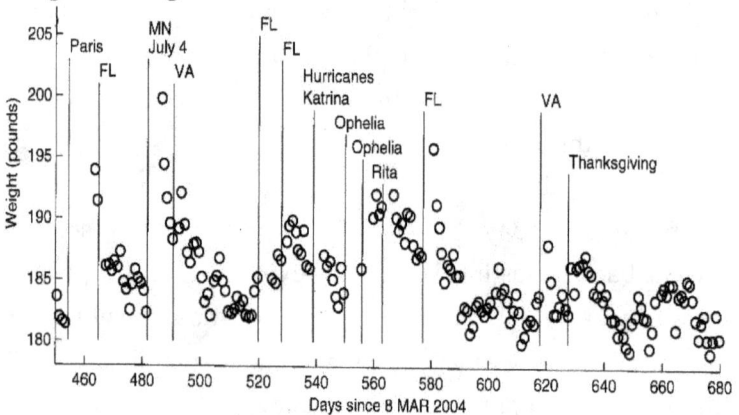

Figure 9

52

I think many people get discouraged by the weight they put on during disruptive periods because they think it's fat. You can't put on fat that quickly, but they say "What's the use?" and just give up trying.

I was surprised my weight increased so little when I went off to fly Hurricane Katrina. Maybe it was because Katrina was a Category 5 when we were flying through it.

By day 680 my weight was fluctuating around an average of about 183 pounds, 44 pounds below where I started. I had not changed my fasting routine or what I ate after the 20-hour fast, but my fat content had stabilized and I was no longer losing weight.

Without any thought or counting or bookkeeping I was consuming exactly the number of calories I needed to maintain my weight. In the evening I ate until I was full, but realized that I was eating less than I did when I began fasting. I think my body just adjusted naturally over time and my food intake reduced gradually. Maybe my stomach shrunk some and it took less to fill it up. Maybe my body recognized I didn't need as much food at my lower weight.

10 RATES FOR GAINING AND LOSING FAT

Figure 10 below provides some insight into the rates for gaining and losing fat. The three plots show my weight variation relative to the starting days of three events. The top plot is referenced to leaving for the 4th of July in Minnesota on day 116. The middle plot is referenced to Christmas on day 292. The bottom plot is referenced to leaving for a business trip to Maryland on day 443.

The Christmas weight gain was documented daily because I was at home. I put on weight at the rate of about 3 pounds per day over the first 3 days. That was about the same rate of weight gain during the 3-day trip to Maryland. Over the trip to Minnesota my weight gain averaged only 1.8 pounds per day.

I suspect that my initial weight gain in Minnesota was also about 3 pounds per day. But after about 3 days my digestive track was at capacity. My rate of weight increase would then slow because the throughput was stabilizing at a higher volume.

When I went back to fasting I quit shoving so much in one end and my weight dropped quickly as things cleared out the other. At the beginning of post-event recovery periods my weight frequently dropped below what would be the new gradual decrease trend and then oscillated about it.

If you consume more calories than you need to maintain your weight you are going to put on fat. But at what rate?

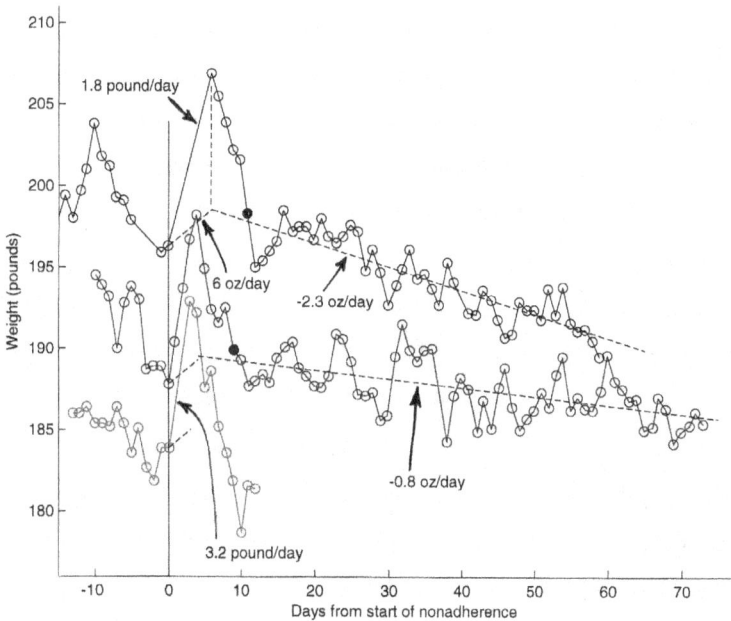

Figure 10

After both the trip to Minnesota and Christmas I had about two months of daily weight measurements that could be used to estimate it.

I least-squares fitted the long dashed straight lines to all the weights to the right, starting from the filled-in circles. I then extended those dashed lines backwards to the left to the day I resumed fasting. I drew the short dashed lines from my weight at the start of the event to join the long dashed line at the time I resumed fasting.

I believe the dashed lines indicate the variation of my body fat over those intervals. When my weight was increasing about 48 ounces (3 pounds) per day, my body fat was only increasing about 6 ounces per day, one-eighth as rapidly.

My fat reduction rate was 2.3 ounces per day after returning from Minnesota and only 0.8 ounces per day after Christmas. But my fat content was about 10 pounds less at Christmas than is was when I went to Minnesota. When you have less fat to lose, you lose it at a slower rate.

After resuming fasting, it typically took about 4 or 5 days for my weight to drop back down to the level from which it would resume a gradual decline. I'm sure most of the excess weight was not fat because I typically lost about 2 pounds a day on the average over those intervals, which was about 8 times faster than my most rapid average fasting weight loss of about a quarter pound per day (Figure 6, graph of days 0 through 120).

I believe the transit time through my digestive track is about a day. So if the excess weight was not fat, why did it take several days to leave? The answer might be fluid retention. I loved salt but had given it up about 20 years earlier when my body quit being able to handle a lot of it and my blood pressure went up. I don't put it on my food and my wife doesn't generally cook with it. I also sweat a lot when I exercise and that purges salt from my body.

When I travel, I eat a lot of fast food. Everybody in Minnesota loves salt and uses a lot of it in cooking. I don't generally exercise much when I'm traveling. So when I'm not fasting, I'm taking in a lot more salt and getting rid of a lot less. Once back home my salt intake is greatly reduced and I'm sweating out a lot of it, but it takes a few days to get back to where I was before I left. I'll leave investigating that hypothesis as a project for some medical researchers.

The dots in Figure 11 below show all of my weights during the 2-year case study. The curve is an exponential decay whose 0.5 decay time constant is 90 days. Exponential decay is the manner in which many natural processes behave. Its characteristic is that it loses exactly the same fraction of its remaining value during any sequence of constant time intervals.

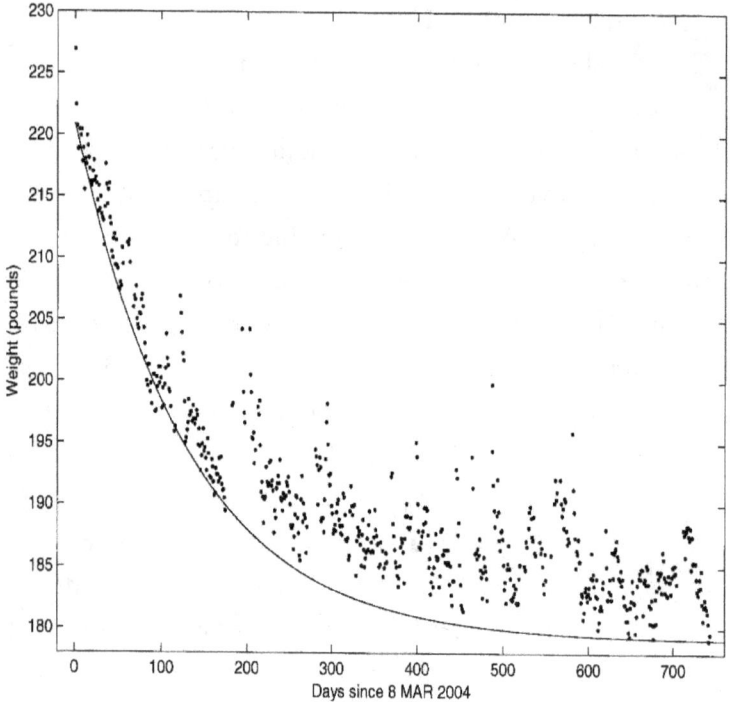

Figure 11

I discounted the rapid initial drop in my weight over the first two days as just clearing out my digestive track and started the decay curve at 221 pounds instead of 227 pounds. I defined the decay curve as if I needed to lose 42 pounds of fat to attain an ideal weight, going from 221 to 179 pounds.

The curve drops 21 pounds (half of what I needed to lose) in the first 90 days. Then it drops 10.5 pounds (half of what I had left to lose) in the next 90 days. It drops 5.25 pounds in the next 90 days and 2.625 pounds in the fourth

90 day interval bringing the total loss to about 39.4 pounds by the end of the first year.

At the beginning of the second year the curve indicates that there is only about 2.6 pounds remaining to be lost and steady state is being approached. The fact that my low weights agree well with the exponential decay curve indicates that was what was happening, despite all the large positive excursions caused by my periods of non-adherence to fasting. I just kept doing the same thing and seamlessly transitioned into an ideal steady state.

11 BODY MASS INDEX

So far, all the weight loss measurements have been in terms of pounds. But if someone who weighs 100 pounds loses 10 pounds, that is more significant than if a 200 pound person loses 10 pounds. Instead of considering the percent of body weight lost, we'll look at the variation of **body mass index** (BMI). Wikipedia, the free web encyclopedia, indicates BMI is a heuristic proxy for human body fat based on an individual's weight and height.

Although BMI, devised in the mid-1800s, does not actually measure the percentage of body fat and makes no allowance for frame size or muscle mass, it is widely used in medicine to categorize people. BMI is computed as an individual's weight in kilograms (kg) divided by the square of their height in meters (m). Any other measurement units can also be used as long as the appropriate multiplicative factor is used to convert the answer to kg/m^2 units. For example,

$$\text{BMI} = \text{weight(kg)} / (\text{height(m)})^2$$
$$= 703 \times \text{weight(pounds)} / (\text{height(inches)})^2$$

A relatively recent study of BMI in the *New England Journal of Medicine* (Calle et al., 1999) which began with over a million participants, found that the lowest rates of death from all causes were for body-mass indexes between 23.5 and 24.9 in men and 22.0 and 23.4 in women, although the relative risks were not significantly elevated for the range of body-mass indexes between 22.0 and 26.4 in men and 20.5 and 24.9 in women. They found that the risk of death increased with increasing BMI in all age groups and for all categories of causes of death.

Figure 12 compares my case study BMI variation with the BMI variations from the Wadden et al. (2005) clinical trial. The horizontal dashed lines indicate the boundaries between BMI values characterizing people as severely obese, moderately obese, overweight, and healthy weight.

The starting average weights of the four Wadden et al. (2005) groups were not very different (232, 234, 238 and 239 pounds) and just 5 to 12 pounds heavier than my 227 pound starting weight. But the average height of each of the four groups was 5 feet 6 inches and my height is 6 feet 3 inches. My height squared was 29% larger than their height squared so my BMI was corresponding lower.

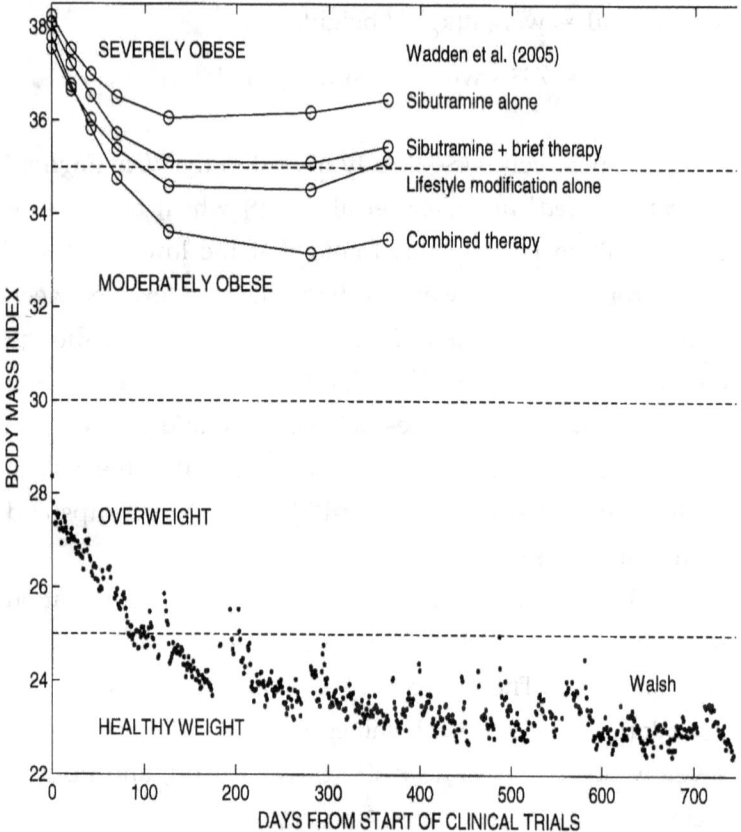

Figure 12

The BMI values of all four groups indicated that they had significantly more fat to lose than I did, but **The 4-Hour Diet** allowed me to shed significantly more weight than any of them. At the end of a year the four Wadden groups were moderately or severely obese and their weight was increasing. At the end of a year, I was nearly at my ideal weight and approaching a steady-state.

LOSING WEIGHT IS NOT ROCKET SCIENCE

12 WILL YOU LOSE HALF YOUR EXCESS FAT IN 90 DAYS?

I lost half my excess fat in the first 90 days, with an average rate of loss of about a quarter pound per day during that interval.   In Figure 13 below I've compared my theoretical exponential decay, drawn as the solid curve, with the weight loss data for the four Wadden et al. (2005) clinical trial groups indicated by the circles connected by the dotted lines.

The Wadden clinical trial was significantly different than the Dansinger et al. (2005) clinical trial of four different diets (Atkins, Ornish, Weight Watchers, Zone).   The Dansinger groups were trying to lose weight with very different diet compositions. The four Wadden groups were trying to lose weight the same way, but with four different aids to help their adherence to the same program.

Since the four Wadden et al. (2005) groups were essentially identical statistically, you could assume that they

63

all began losing weight at the same rate, indicated by the exponential decay. Then each group drifted up and away from that curve as their adherence diminished.

In the first Wadden weight measurements after the start of the clinical trial (day 21), the "Sibutramine alone" group was already lagging significantly, having lost two pounds less than the "combined therapy" group. The other two groups had lost a pound less than that best group.

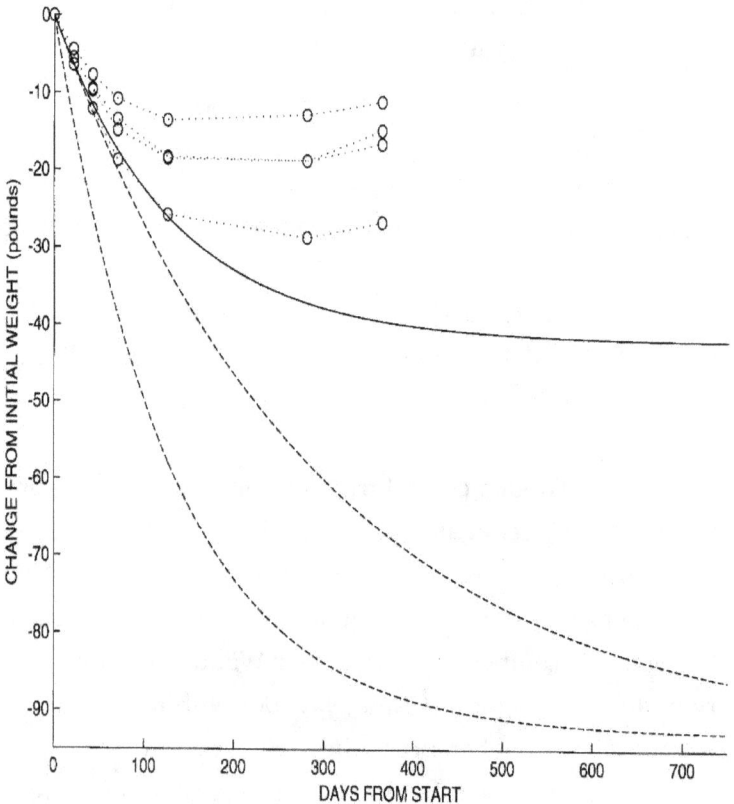

Figure 13

By day 126, three of the four Wadden groups were well above my exponential decay curve, but the best performing group was right on it. By the next set of measurements (day 280) all the Wadden groups were above my exponential decay curve.

A benefit of having a large group in a clinical trial is that the participants have different things going on in their lives. Their individual weight fluctuations, so apparent in my daily record, will occur at different times. On the day they are weighed, some of the 60 people in each group will be deviating above their trend line while others will be deviating below it. The group average weight will very accurately indicate the group trend.

At first glance it seems like the best performing group lost adherence after day 126, but if you look closely you will see that the best Wadden group weight is actually below my exponential decay curve at day 70. I think that group actually began to lose adherence even earlier than that.

With an average weight of 236 pounds and an average height of 5 feet 6 inches, the Wadden groups would have needed to lose 93 pounds to achieve a BMI of 23. My 42 pound excess fat weight loss followed an exponential decay, which meant that as my excess fat diminished, my rate of loss also diminished. When I lost 10 pounds I only had 32 pounds left to lose. When the Wadden group lost 10 pounds they still had 83 pounds remaining to lose, so their rate of loss should have diminished less than mine because their status had changed less than mine.

The first dashed curve below the solid curve in Figure 13 is an exponential decay that has the same initial rate of loss as the solid curve at the beginning, but ends 93 pounds below the starting weight instead of 42 pounds below it. When you compare the best performing Wadden group to that dashed curve it begins to diverge after day 42. The 0.5 decay time for that curve is 200 days instead of 90 days. If the best Wadden group had maintained the adherence they had in the first six weeks, their weight loss would probably have followed that dashed curve.

The lower dashed curve is an exponential decay which drops 93 pounds, but with a 90-day 0.5 decay time, the same as the solid curve. The steep curve has an initial rate of loss of 0.7 pounds per day, almost 5 pounds per week. That kind of loss is certainly attainable when you consider the rates of loss in evidence on The Biggest Loser, but most people would not sustain the level of effort required. And that rate of loss might not be advisable.

On the web, I found an article written by Edward Wyatt ("On 'The Biggest Loser,' Health Can Take Back Seat," published 24 November 2009, **The New York Times**). Wyatt said that medical professionals generally advise against losing more than about two pounds a week. He indicated that more rapid weight loss can cause many medical problems, including a weakening of the heart muscle, irregular heartbeat, and dangerous reductions in potassium and electrolytes.

The initial rate of weight loss for the exponential decay curve (Figure 11 and solid curve in Figure 13) that provided the lower asymptote for my weights over my 2-year case study is 2.2 pounds a week. So not only did **The 4-Hour Diet** allow me to achieve my ideal weight, it achieved it in an ideal way.

After doing this analysis, I looked around the web and found that I was not the first person to recognize that fasting weight loss followed an exponential decay curve. Gilbert B. Forbes, M.D., published a similar analysis in *The American Journal of Clinical Nutrition* more than 40 years ago. There was one significant difference. The technique Forbes studied was not sustainable.

Forbes (1970) used data from several different clinical studies. The most statistically significant group was 9 men who were so excessively obese that they were willing to undergo supervised starvation with their weights being measured daily so the researchers could determine how that method of weight loss would affect their body composition.

Forbes did not indicate their heights, but the average initial weight of the 9 men was 314 pounds. If their average height was 5' 9", which was the average height of men in 1970, then the average BMI of the group would have been 46 and they would have to lose 157 pounds to attain a BMI of 23.

Forbes fit the sum of two exponential decay curves to the variation of each participant's total weight, not to an estimate of their excess fat as I did in my case study. The fast exponential decay curve accounted for about 4% of their total weight. The slow exponential decay curve accounted for the other 96%. The fast exponential decay curve had a starting value of 12 pounds and a 0.5 decay time of 2.8 days. That is similar to the rapid weight losses I experienced each time I resumed fasting after an interruption.

After the initial week when the fast decay curve value became negligible, the Forbes slow exponential decay curve was in excellent agreement with the variation in total weight of the group. It had an average 0.5 decay time of 190 days, very similar to the 200 days I had projected for the four Wadden groups, but the initial rate of weight loss was 7.5 pounds per week.

Projecting the Forbes slow exponential decay curve forward in time demonstrates how extreme and un-sustainable the starving technique is. At the end of two years the curve approaches a total weight of twenty pounds, the average weight of an adult human skeleton, and the participants would have long since perished. They had no caloric input. Their decay curve indicates that their entire bodies were wasting away. The starving trials of the 9 men were terminated after 50 to 125 days.

Since **The 4-Hour Diet** allowed me unrestricted eating during a 4-hour interval every day, my entire body was not wasting away. Twenty-hour fasting could be continued indefinitely because my total weight stabilized at an ideal value, not that of a skeleton. Without changing anything, I attained and then maintained an ideal weight.

Table 1 below will save you from some arithmetic. I plugged numbers into the equation for Body Mass Index in the previous chapter to find the relationship between height and weight for someone with a BMI of 23. As I indicated earlier, BMI does not make allowance for frame size, or having more than usual muscle mass, the situation for many athletes. But if you take the weights in Table 1 to be the ideal and assume weighing more is due to excess fat, the numbers might provide a general sense of the amount of excess fat you may have to lose to achieve your ideal weight.

The final graph, Figure 14, is my projection of how your excess fat might decrease over time, depending on how much you had when you began. I generated the curves by assuming that everyone's initial rate of weight loss would be 2.2 pounds a week.

Table 1

Height (feet, inches)	Weight (pounds)	Height (feet, inches)	Weight (pounds)	Height (feet, inches)	Weight (pounds)
4' 6"	95.4	5' 3"	129.9	6'	169.6
4' 7"	99.0	5' 4"	134.0	6' 1"	174.4
4' 8"	102.6	5' 5"	138.2	6' 2"	179.2
4' 9"	106.3	5' 6"	142.5	6' 3"	184.0
4' 10"	110.1	5' 7"	146.9	6' 4"	189.0
4' 11"	113.9	5' 8"	151.3	6' 5"	194.0
5'	117.8	5' 9"	155.8	6' 6"	199.0
5' 1"	121.7	5' 10"	160.3	6' 7"	204.2
5' 2"	125.8	5' 11"	164.9	6' 8"	209.4

That was my rate of loss when I had 42 pounds of fat to lose. It was also the initial rate of loss for the people in the Wadden et al. (2005) study, and they had about 93 pounds of fat to lose. I assumed that the excess fat would decrease exponentially, so the rate of loss would decrease as the remaining fat decreased.

You would have to acquire weight loss data from people following the program who began with many different excess fat amounts to verify the curves experimentally. But I think the curves might provide you with a useful perspective for what you might expect in your own case study.

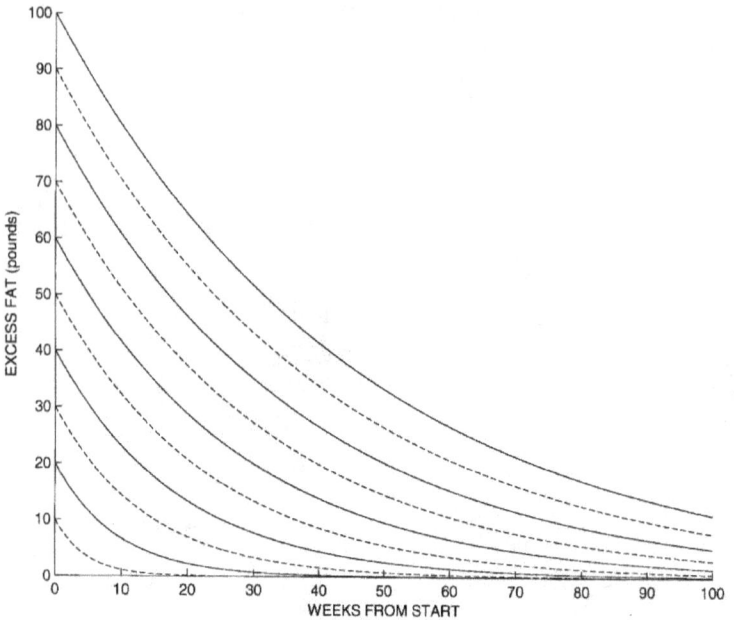

Figure 14

The curves indicate a reasonable rate of weight loss. For example, the curve starting at 90 pounds of excess fat indicates a loss of more than 40 pounds in 6 months, and about 65 pounds by the end of the first year.

In contrast, each of the four groups in the Wadden et al. (2005) study had about 93 pounds of fat to lose and the best-performing group lost less than 30 pounds over the entire year.

The curves can also put some of **The 8-Hour Diet** and **The Fast-5 Diet** numbers in perspective. Herring indicated that someone on **The Fast-5 Diet** could start losing a pound a week and maintain that loss rate for a year, losing 52 pounds if they had that much to lose. If you start losing only a pound a week, that rate will diminish over time and you won't lose 52 pounds in a year. My curves above indicate that someone with 52 pounds of excess fat to lose would start losing 2.2 pounds per week and lose a total of about 46 pounds over the first year.

Six of the seven success stories in **The 8-Hour Diet** highlight individuals who lost 12 to 20 pounds in 6 weeks. We don't know how often those people weighed themselves. Since my case study shows that your weight can fluctuate several pounds in a few days, the people might well have reported the lowest number their weight attained within a day or so of day 42, rather than averaging their daily weights over 7 days centered on day 42.

If a person's rate of weight loss were constant at 2.2

pounds per week, they would lose 13.2 pounds in 6 weeks. But since weight loss follows an exponential decay, the less excess fat you have to begin with, the faster the rate of loss will decrease. Someone with less excess fat to begin with will lose less weight over a 6 week period than someone with a lot. Table 2 below indicates what the Figure 14 graphs suggest would be the amount of fat lost in 6 weeks as a function of the starting excess fat.

The person who reported losing 20 pounds in six weeks on **The 8-Hour Diet** initially weighed 315 pounds and had about 140 pounds of excess fat to lose. I lost about 6 pounds in the first two days that I didn't count in the exponential decay. That, plus the 12.6 pounds from the exponential decay, adds up to a weight loss of about 18.6 pounds, which is close to the 20 pounds he reported. And he probably started with more in his digestive track than I did.

Table 2

EXCESS FAT (pounds)	FAT LOST IN 6 WEEKS (pounds)
10	7.3
20	9.7
40	10.7
80	12.2
140	12.6

13 GENERAL COMMENTS

It takes much less to maintain fat than it does muscle. A recent study of resting metabolic rates (Wang et al. 2011) confirmed that the values published by Elia (1992) were valid and not subject to gender influences for the non-elderly (age 20 - 49 years) and non-obese (BMI 18.5 – 29.9). Even when resting, skeletal muscle burns calories at three times the rate for fat. Once you have eaten too much over a long time and have a high percentage of fat, you don't have to eat much more than other people to maintain it.

When you start losing weight, will you just be losing the fat? While I'm cooling down after finishing the treadmill I generally do a half dozen weight-machine exercises, most of them for the upper body. So I'm confident my entire weight loss was fat. There is a range of opinions on the web about the general composition of weight loss during dieting. The consensus seems to be that the body will burn more fat than muscle because it needs the muscle to go find more food.

Gilbert B. Forbes, M.D., author of the book *Human body composition: growth, aging, nutrition and activity* as well as 150 articles and 45 book chapters, indicated that in most situations involving a significant loss of weight, both body fat and fat-free body mass will be reduced (Forbes, 2000). The relative contribution of each to the total weight reduction is influenced by the initial body fat content. The higher your initial body fat content, the higher the percentage of weight loss that will be fat.

If you are not exercising and lose 30 pounds, some of it will have been muscle. If you then put 30 pounds back on without exercising, it will be mostly fat. So you will be more fat than when you started and your metabolism will be lower. That's the danger of yo-yo dieting. If you cycle your weight several times without exercising you will be progressively worse off.

Why not hedge your bets? Do a few body-weight exercises in the morning. Pushups require very little time. You can start doing them from your knees and eventually switch to your toes. They will strengthen, tone and increase the muscle mass in your arms, chest and shoulders. They also strengthen the core muscles around your midsection. Take a walk at noon during the time you save by not eating lunch.

My two-year case study involved only one healthy adult (me) and had no medical supervision. I did fine, but that's no guarantee everyone else would. What would happen if you were diabetic? Or pregnant or nursing? Or a child? Or any number of other things? I don't know.

People should be certain that fasting is not contraindicated for their circumstances. It would not be advisable for anyone to impose this regimen on someone else. People should be free to make their own evaluation of their situation in consultation with their health care provider when deciding whether to participate, and to assess their status as time goes on.

If your weight is stable, you are ingesting exactly the number of calories needed to maintain it. If you want to weigh less, you need to eat less. I've demonstrated that fasting for a 20-hour interval each day will do that automatically without changing the composition of your diet or putting any restriction on your consumption when you do eat.

In the afternoon I'm aware my stomach is empty, but it's not distracting. I can easily go until 8 PM without eating. What is very difficult is to eat a little and stop.

Although **The 4-Hour Diet** is not physically difficult, you will have to overcome your habit of reaching for food during the day. Initially, you can pursue fasting one day at a time. If you can just make it until 6 PM without eating, you can relax and enjoy yourself without guilt.

It may take you a couple of failed attempts to get going, but that doesn't cost you anything. Once you've done it for a few days, it's easy. You won't get hunger pangs and you'll be able to pass up any offer of food.

Stay rested. Fatigue is the enemy of discipline.

Don't get dehydrated. Drink all the water you need. It has no calories.

It should be apparent why **The 4-Hour Diet** is better than **The 8-Hour Diet**. Once you haven't consumed any calories for 16 hours, you're burning fat and you won't get hunger pangs because your blood sugar is low. At that point, continuing the fast for another 4 hours will significantly increase your fat burn and reduce your caloric intake when you do eat.

If you have only a 4-hour interval for eating, it will be difficult to consume as many calories as you would have distributed throughout the day. There is no time for your stomach to empty out and fill up again. If the eating interval is 8 hours, that is not the case.

That is not to say that restricting eating to an 8-hour interval will not be of benefit. That is also not to say that if you eat during an 8-hour interval only three days a week, it won't be of any benefit. It just won't be of as much benefit. Why not try to maximize your benefit? It takes little additional effort to fast the extra 4 hours, or to fast 7 days a week if you have no disruptions.

It is important to realize that fasting 20 hours a day is significantly more than 25% better than fasting 16 hours a day. Marathon runners don't hit the wall when they wake up. And they don't hit the wall in the first mile of the race. They have expended a lot of energy before they have only fat left to keep them going.

With a 16 hour fast, you certainly have less than 8 hours of maximum fat burning. As you begin the fasting interval, your body is digesting and utilizing the food just taken in. And your energy expenditure is significantly reduced while you're asleep. When you wake and increase your energy demand, your body prefers to use the glycogen stored in your liver and muscles before it goes after the fat. So if you increase your fasting interval by 4 hours, you'll probably increase your fat burn by 50%.

An important recommendation of **The 4-Hour Diet** is that your 4 hours of unrestricted eating should be your last 4 hours awake. If you ate only during your first 4 hours awake, the weight loss would be the same. But you wouldn't stick with the program. After that first 4 hours, you'd be awake for 12 hours with no caloric intake, assuming you sleep 8 hours. Your blood sugar level spiked by all that initial eating would plummet, you'd get hunger pangs and not be able to concentrate on anything but getting something else to eat. And you might have trouble getting to sleep with your stomach empty. If you set the eating interval from noon to 4 PM, you'd still get hungry before you went to bed. I'll bet even many of the people using **The 8-Hour Diet** end up cheating before they go to bed.

The daily weight measurements and analysis of my

case study provide significantly more encouragement than other weight-loss programs which just try to convince you to use their technique without providing a realistic indication of how you can expect your weight to vary.

My daily weights demonstrate you can eat the same foods you always have, live with all the world's disruptions, and still accomplish your goals. Just fast whenever you can and your body will take care of the rest automatically.

It is important to recognize that my daily weight measurements show that even if you are on your way to an ideal weight, your apparent weight loss will not be monotonic. The fluctuations in your weight that a scale indicates will always be large compared to your trend, even if you are fasting every day. But be confident that if you are fasting every day, you will be burning fat and your intrinsic weight will be decreasing monotonically.

If you have a lot to lose, you have to make a long-term commitment to be successful. I've demonstrated that you can stick to **The 4-Hour Diet** for years.

You don't have to give up socializing while you're fasting. When my wife and I go to one of our community morning coffee get-togethers, there are loads of delicious pastries around, but I'm not tempted. If anyone asks me why I'm not eating, I tell them about **The 4-Hour Diet**. They don't feel awkward and it just becomes an additional interesting topic of conversation.

The 4-Hour Diet will work whether or not you

record your weight daily. But it is important to document your effort, even by doing something as simple as putting a check mark on a calendar each day you fast. That will give you a real sense of accomplishment and motivate you to get that next check mark.

You can attain and maintain your ideal weight. You'll feel better, have more confidence, improve your health and appearance, and be the envy of your friends.

If this information has been helpful, please write a brief customer review at amazon.com. Thank you. Good luck and good health.

If you want to read an inspirational book, get my wife's memoir, **RIVER CITY a nurse's year in Vietnam**, available at Amazon.com, either as an ebook for $2.99 or a trade paperback for $14.95. Pat volunteered for Vietnam as a civilian nurse in 1967 to care for Vietnamese caught in the crossfire. She lived unprotected in downtown Danang and worked incredibly hard, never expecting to fall in love, or the Tet Offensive.

Pat chronicles the dedication, self sacrifice, trials and triumphs of combat medicine in a primitive Vietnamese hospital where most of their medical supplies were diverted to the Black Market. Paramount Pictures optioned her story for Cher the year she won Best Actress. But the project went into turnaround when they couldn't get a good script.

If you want to know what it was like for people returning from Vietnam with Post-Traumatic Stress Disorder (PTSD), get **CEMETERY PICNICS**, Pat's novel available at amazon.com as an ebook for $2.99. You can read the first several chapters of either book at amazon.com using their ebook "Look Inside" feature.

At **patriciawalsh.com** you can watch brief excerpts from **The Other Angels**, a documentary Pat made about her medical team. It won the People's Choice Award at the Denver International Film Festival, aired across the country on PBS, was named Booklist Editors' Choice by the American Library Association, and won a Gracie and the Grand Award from American Women in Radio and Television.

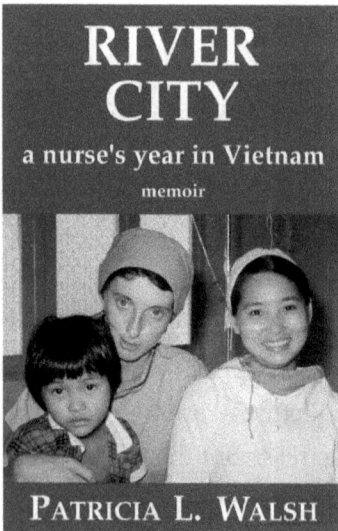

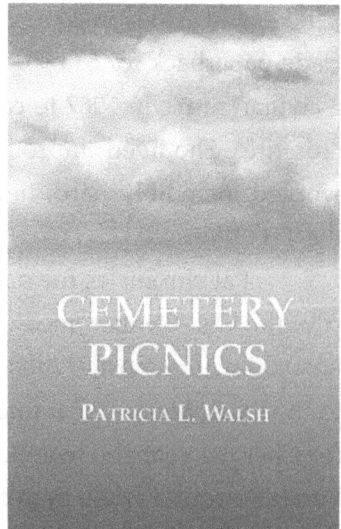

RIVER CITY
a nurse's year in Vietnam
memoir

PATRICIA L. WALSH

CEMETERY PICNICS
PATRICIA L. WALSH

14 REFERENCES

Calle, E. E., M. J. Thun, J. M. Petrelli, C. Rodriguez, C. W. Heath, Jr., (1999): Body-Mass Index and Mortality in a Prospective Cohort of U.S. Adults. *New England Journal of Medicine*, 341:1097-1105.

Daly, M. E., C. Vale, M. Walker, A. Littlefield, K. G. Alberti, J. C. Mathers, (1998): Acute effects on insulin sensitivity and diurnal metabolic profiles of a high-sucrose compared with a high-starch diet. *The American Journal of Clinical Nutrition*, 67:1186-96.

Dansinger, M. L., J. A. Gleason, J. L. Griffith, H. P. Selker, E. J. Schaefer, (2005): Comparison of the Atkins, Ornish, Weight Watchers, and Zone diets for weight loss and heart disease risk reduction: a randomized trial. *Journal of the American Medical Association*, 293:43-53.

Davies, P., (2000): Inside the Hurricane, face to face

with nature's deadliest storms. *Henry Holt and Company, LLC*, 264 pages.

Elia, M. (1992): Organ and tissue contribution to metabolic rate. In: Energy Metabolism: Tissue Determinants and Cellular Corollaries. J. M. Kinney and H. N. Tucker, editors. *Raven Press*, New York, 61-80.

Forbes, G. B., (1970): Weight loss during fasting: implications for the obese. *The American Journal of Clinical Nutrition*, 23(9):1212-1219.

Forbes, G. B., (1987): Human body composition: growth, aging, nutrition and activity. *Springer*, 350 pages.

Forbes, G. B., (2000): Body fat content influences the body composition response to nutrition and exercise. *Annals of the New York Academy of Sciences*, May, 904:359-365.

Herring, B. W., (2005): The Fast-5 Diet and the Fast-5 Lifestyle. *Fast-5 LLC*, 58 pages.

Hofmekler, O., (2003): The Warrior Diet : Switch on your biological powerhouse for high energy, explosive strength, and a leaner, harder body. *Blue Snake Books*, 312 pages.

Jampolis, M., (2007): The No-Time to Lose Diet: The busy person's guide to permanent weight loss. *Nelson Books*, 226 pages.

Ludwig, D. S., M. I. Friedman (2014): Always Hungry? Here's Why. *The New York Times*, Sunday Review, May18.

Ng, M., T. Fleming, M. Robertson, B. Thomson, N. Graetz, C. Margono, E. C. Mullany, S. Biryukov, C. Abbafati, S. F. Abera, J. P. Abraham, N. M. E. Abu-Rmeileh, and 128 additional authors (2014): Global, regional, and national prevalence of overweight and obesity in children and adults during 1980–2013: a systematic analysis for the Global Burden of Disease Study 2013. *The Lancet*, Early Online Publication, 29 May 2014, doi:10.1016/S0140-6736(14)60460-8.

Ogden, C. L., M. D. Carroll, B. K. Kit, K. M. Flegal, (2014): Prevalence of Chldhood and Adult Obesity in the United States, 2011-2012. *Journal of the American Medical Association*, *JAMA*. 2014;311(8):806-814. Doi:10.1001/jama .2014.732.

Smith, I. K., (2013): SHRED: THE REVOLUTION-ARY DIET. *St. Martin's Press*, 268 pages.

Wadden, T. A., R. I. Berkowitz, L. G. Wombie, D. B. Sarwer, S. Phelan, R. K. Cato, L. A. Hesson, S. Y. Osei, R. Kaplan, A. J. Stunkard, (2005): Randomized trial of lifestyle modification and pharmacotherapy for obesity. *New England Journal of Medicine*, 353:2111-2120.

Walsh, E. J., (2006): The fast way to lose weight. *American Journal of Bariatric Medicine*, 21-3:10-13.

Wang Z, Z. Ying, A. Bosy-westphal, J. Zhang, M. Heller, W. Later, S. B. Heymsfield, M. J. Muller, (2011): Evaluation of specific metabolic rates of major organs and tissues: comparison between men and women. *American Journal of Human Biology*, 23(3):333-338.

Zinczenko, D., P. Moore, (2013): The 8-Hour Diet: Watch the pounds disappear without watching what you eat!. *Rodale Books*, 288 pages.